# OUTSMARTING
# DIABETES

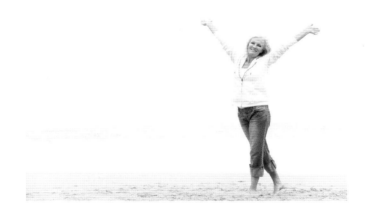

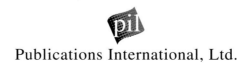

Publications International, Ltd.

Editor and contributing writer: Juliane Bylica

Contributing writers: Dana Armstrong, R.D., C.D.E.; Timothy Gower; Allen Bennett King, M.D., F.A.C.P.; Gary Scheiner, M.S., C.D.E.

Louis Weber, CEO
Publications International, Ltd.
7373 North Cicero Avenue
Lincolnwood, Illinois 60712

ISBN: 978-1-4508-8686-4

Manufactured in China.

8 7 6 5 4 3 2 1

# Contents

# Introduction

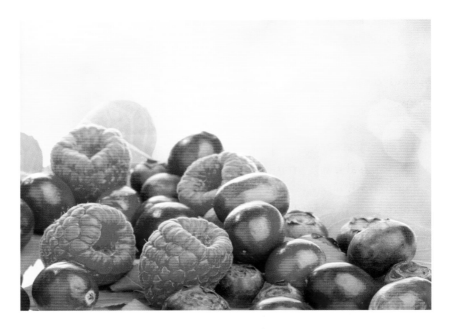

Managing diabetes is a big, complex, ongoing job. Unlike most other medical conditions, the disease affects every major organ system in the body. Especially if you've only received a diagnosis recently, the task of managing your disease can seem daunting. In *Outsmarting Diabetes*, we give you some tools to tackle the task. Make no mistake: Living an active, independent life is possible with diabetes.

# Taking Control

You don't need to feel trapped by your diabetes. When you understand your disease and become an active participant in your own care, you'll feel liberated. When you know and use the tools available to you, you'll find yourself feeling better, enjoying better blood sugar control, and lowering your risk of complications.

# Finding Information

One tool at your disposal is information. Faced with a health problem, we sometimes want to bury our head in the sand. It's easier to avoid thinking about potential problems we may encounter, or lifestyle changes we may need to adopt. But the more you know, the better your chances at avoiding those potential problems. Knowing the facts about diabetes and being honest with yourself about your own health sets you up to manage your health in the most effective ways.

In *Outsmarting Diabetes*, you'll find plenty of information. In the opening chapters, we cover the basics of the disease, explaining its causes, its variations, and its symptoms in terms a layperson can understand. You'll find information on the costs of unregulated high blood sugar, and the benefits you'll see when your blood sugar is under control. And you'll find ideas for how to assemble a care team that will help you manage the disease.

# Blood Sugar Regulation

In chapter 4, you'll find information on the details of blood sugar regulation. More than most other medical conditions, diabetes demands that you take charge of your own care. The idea of testing your blood each day—maybe even several times a day—can be intimidating, but it's a crucial part of managing your care. If you've been wondering what supplies you'll need to test your blood sugar levels, what your numbers should be, or what your "A1c level" means, turn to this chapter.

# Lifestyle Changes

Anyone who goes into a checkout line at the supermarket or looks at the array of magazines in a waiting room knows that there are a lot of suggestions out there for ways to lead a healthy lifestyle, from the newest trend diet to the latest exercise fad. Sifting out the suggestions you want to follow can prove difficult, and having diabetes only makes it more complicated.

However, the lifestyle changes you can make, including changes to your diet and exercise routine, are some of your most powerful tools in managing diabetes. In chapters 5 through 7, you'll find tried-and-tested information about how to balance your food intake, suggestions for starting and maintaining an exercise program, and tips for lowering your stress levels.

## The Scoop on Medication and Insulin

Not all people with diabetes take medication or insulin, but these too can be a powerful tool in your arsenal. While you'll need to discuss the specifics of your situation with your doctor and the rest of your care team to learn what, if any, medications are right for you, chapter 8 provides an overview into the current available medications, including their strengths and potential side effects. Chapter 9 goes in depth about insulin therapy—if your doctor has mentioned insulin therapy as a possibility, read this chapter to get a better idea of what questions you should ask and what factors you should take into account.

## Prevention and Troubleshooting

Diabetes can come with a host of health complications. In the book's final chapters, you'll find material on preventing these complications,

or handling them if they occur. Hypoglycemic episodes are one of the most common problems resulting from diabetes, and they are covered in-depth in Chapter 10. In the final chapter, you'll find information on how to protect your eyes, feet, and skin, so you can know what symptoms to watch out for, derailing health issues as soon as they start.

## Three Keys to Treating, Delaying, or Preventing Complications

**Education**
Learn as much as you can about diabetes.
**Early Detection**
Learn the signs and symptoms of potential problems
**Regular Office Visits**
Set up a schedule and stick to it!

# Diabetes: A Brief History

Papyrus documents unearthed in Egypt that appear to be medical records, dating back to 1552 B.C., mention patients with symptoms that sound like diabetes. In the first century AD, a doctor named Aretaeus in what is now Turkey) noticed that some of his patients were weak, constantly thirsty, and needed to urinate a lot. It seemed to him that something was causing fluids to be drawn out of their bodies, so he called the condition diabetes, which is the Greek word for "siphon."

An 11th century Arab physician, Avicenna, fine-tuned the diagnosis when he discovered that people with diabetes produced what he called "wonderfully sweet" urine. How did he scientifically verify that? Yes: He tasted it.

Centuries later, a similarly brave and selfless British physician detected notes of clover in the urine of his diabetic patients and coined the phrase diabetes mellitus, adding the Latin word for "honey sweet." Mind you, all this taste testing served a purpose. Doctors eventually learned that the sweetness of diabetics' urine came from sugar. A theory developed that the diabetic body produces too much of the sweet stuff, in the form of glucose, which is flushed out in the urine.

Doctors eventually began to suspect that the culprit was a malfunctioning organ. But which one? The kidneys came under scrutiny first, then the liver. However, in 1889 a pair of enterprising scientists found the truth when they removed a dog's pancreas, only to return the next day and discover that the previously house-trained pooch had peed all over his cage. Noting that people with diabetes have a hard time holding their water, the doctors suspected that the pancreas might play some role in controlling blood sugar. Testing the dog's urine confirmed their suspicion: It was loaded with glucose.

Until then, scientists thought that the pancreas manufactured digestive enzymes and not much else. It soon became clear, however, that when the pancreas was missing or malfunctioning, glucose built up in the blood, resulting in diabetes. So maybe the problem wasn't that the body made too much glucose. Maybe the pancreas made too little of something else.

At last, scientists figured out the role played by cells in the pancreas called islets of Langerhans (named for the man who discovered them). In the early 1920s, other researchers showed that these pancreatic cells make a substance that "unlocks" cells throughout the rest of the body, allowing glucose to enter so it can be used as a source of energy. That all-important hormone is insulin.

# Understand the Problem

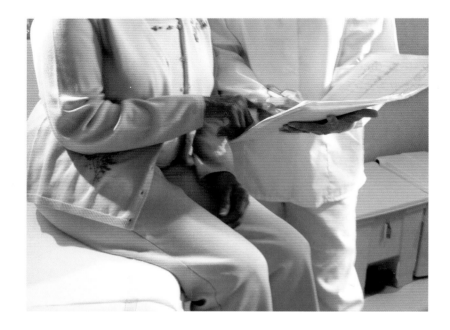

If you want to get control of your diabetes, you need to get to know your disease. This first chapter provides an overview—what diabetes is, how it develops, and other important information—that will get you acquainted with what's going on in your body so that you can manage your condition as effectively as possible.

# What Is Diabetes?

In simplest terms, diabetes is a problem with energy production. (In medical terms, it's a metabolic disorder.) If you have diabetes, your body can't efficiently use glucose, which is the body's main source of energy. It's not that you lack glucose. Unless you're fasting or on the All-Beef-and-Butter diet, you've got plenty of glucose in your system from the carbohydrates in the food you eat. The problem is getting the glucose into your cells, which need it to produce energy. The cells, for reasons we will explain, bar the glucose from entering. As a result, the glucose floats around in your bloodstream, slowly damaging everything in its path.

# Fueling Up

Let's back up for a minute. To understand where the diabetic body goes awry, it will help to know how the body is supposed to process food and use it for energy. Humans can burn fat and protein as fuel, and in fact, muscles prefer to use fatty acids. But for the body as a whole, the preferred source of energy is carbohydrates, which it breaks down into a sugar called glucose. Glucose is the only fuel the brain can use.

Your seventh-grade teacher probably explained that carbohydrates are sugars and starches found in fruits, vegetables, and grain products, such as bread and rice. While that's true, it's hardly the whole picture, since soda pop, pizza, potato chips, cupcakes, and virtually any other form of junk food you can think of are also packed with carbs. Clearly, some carbohydrate-rich foods are healthier than others. But once food has been digested, your body can't tell whether a carbohydrate came from a banana or a candy bar. Regardless of their source, all carbohydrates become glucose in the body.

When you eat a meal that contains carbohydrate, your body converts the carbohydrate into glucose during the digestion process. In a flash, the glucose

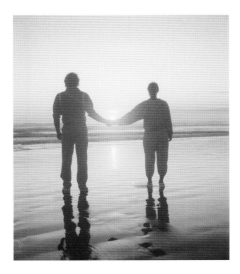

enters the bloodstream—which is why glucose is referred to as *blood sugar*—and is quickly absorbed by the body's cells.

Some of it is immediately used for energy, while the rest is placed into short-term storage—in the form of glycogen—primarily in the liver and muscle tissues. If you eat way more carbohydrate than you need for immediate energy and short-term reserves, your body will convert the glucose into fat, which it ships off for long-term storage, usually in the belly, butt, and thighs. Likewise, if your body's immediate and short-term energy needs are covered by the carbs in your meal, the fat from the food will be sent to long-term storage.

If glucose could simply slip into your body's cells on its own, there would be no such thing as diabetes, and you could be out working in the garden or playing with the kids (or watching reruns) instead of reading this book. However, glucose needs assistance from a hormone called insulin, which acts like a doorman, unlocking cells so that glucose can enter and be used as fuel.

Insulin production is regulated by the pancreas, an organ tucked under the stomach that is five to six inches long and looks sort of like a squished snail. The pancreas actually produces a pair of hormones that regulate glucose levels in the blood. Hormones are the body's expediters, zipping around from one organ to another, making things happen. When the level of glucose in the blood begins to rise, the pancreas cranks out insulin to help get the glucose into the cells. When blood sugar levels drop too low, the pancreas produces glucagon, a hormone that travels to the liver with orders to convert some glycogen back

## By the Numbers

Here are some quick facts about diabetes, according to the latest available National Diabetes Fact Sheet:

- 25.8 million Americans—8.3 percent of the population—have diabetes (diagnosed and undiagnosed cases).
- 7 million Americans have diabetes but don't know it.
- 11.3 percent of Americans aged 20 years and older have diabetes.
- 1.9 million new cases of diabetes are diagnosed each year in Americans aged 20 years and older.

into glucose and release it into the blood. With these two hormones, the pancreas helps you maintain a stable level of blood sugar.

# You Just Can't Get Good Help

As mentioned earlier, people with diabetes don't lack for glucose—they have plenty of the stuff. The problem is with the doormen. In people with type 1 diabetes, these gatekeepers never show up for work. In people with type 2 diabetes, the doormen arrive for duty but can't figure out how to unlock the gate. The result is the same in both cases: Glucose can't enter cells.

Here is a closer look at the main forms of diabetes.

# Type 1 Diabetes

If you have type 1 diabetes, the chances are pretty good that you have known it for a long time: Half of all people diagnosed with type 1 diabetes are younger than 20 years old. In fact, type 1 diabetes used to be called juvenile-onset diabetes, back before doctors realized that the condition can actually strike people of any age. Another name sometimes used is insulin-dependent diabetes, since virtually all folks with type 1 require injections of

the crucial hormone. Only about 5 to 10 percent of all people with diabetes have type 1, making it far less common than type 2 diabetes.

Type 1 diabetes begins with a glitch in the immune system, the body's defense against bacteria, viruses, and other unwanted invaders that roam around your body, trying to make you sick. The immune system is a complex network of vessels, fluids, white blood cells, and special proteins called antibodies that patrol your innards, looking for things that don't belong. When your immune system detects a germ or anything else that it doesn't recognize as belonging to the body, it fires off white blood cells and antibodies to engulf and destroy the intruder.

Unfortunately, in some people the immune system is guilty of friendly fire. It mistakes perfectly innocent and otherwise healthy body tissue for an enemy invader, attacking it with an onslaught of voracious immune cells. Depending on what part of the body your immune system attacks, the result can be one of many autoimmune diseases, which include rheumatoid arthritis, lupus, thyroiditis, and, yes, type 1 diabetes.

If you have type 1 diabetes, your immune system unleashed an assault on the cells in your pancreas that make insulin, known as beta cells. As your beta cells died off, your insulin production slowed down and may even have stopped. Without sufficient insulin to control the amount of glucose in your blood, your blood glucose levels began to rise, causing symptoms of diabetes. The symptoms likely included:

- an unquenchable thirst. No matter how much liquid you guzzled, you still felt parched.
- a frequent need to urinate. Your bladder likely felt ready to burst whether or not you were gulping down fluids.
- increased hunger. You may have felt ravenous despite having recently eaten.
- sudden weight loss. Now you might be thinking, *Do you mean I get to eat like a pig and lose a few pounds at the same time? Sign me up!* Not so fast. Type 1 diabetes causes weight loss because your body is more or less devouring itself, which is not a good thing.
- unexplained fatigue. You probably felt drained no matter how much sleep and rest you got and how much food you ate.

It's easy to see from these diverse symptoms just how important insulin is to the proper functioning of the human body. When glucose has no way of entering your cells, the sugary substance starts to build up in the blood. Your body has to pull water out of the blood (increasing thirst) so that it can get rid of the excess glucose in the urine (which explains the frequent trips to the restroom). Your cells are screaming for fuel (triggering the "Let's order another pizza!" instinct in your brain). While they're waiting for more glucose, your cells switch to alternate sources of energy, so the body starts to run on fat. That's the reason you lose weight, but it's kind of like burning the furniture in the fireplace when you can't pay the heating bill. And the combination of high blood glucose levels and dehydration makes you feel tired.

Burning fat all day instead of glucose isn't just inefficient; it can be life threatening if it goes on too long. As your body breaks down fat to use as energy, it produces leftover products called ketones. Does that word ring a bell? You may have heard of ketones and ketosis (the accumulation of ketones when fat is burned for energy) if you have tried the carbohydrate-hating Atkins diet. In his book *Dr. Atkins' Diet Revolution*, the late Robert Atkins, M.D., claimed that ketosis is "a signal for rejoicing...a state devoutly to be desired...." Why? Because, according to Atkins, it means you're burning unsightly fat and shedding flab!

Obesity experts disagree whether intentionally triggering ketosis is a safe and effective weight-loss method, but many diet doctors insist that some people lose weight on the Atkins plan not because of metabolic trickery but because it's just another low-calorie diet. (Studies have failed to show that it's superior to other weight-loss approaches in the long run.)

What's not up for debate is whether high levels of ketones are dangerous for the person with diabetes. Normally, these compounds pass harmlessly from your system into your urine to be excreted. But when carbohydrates are entirely removed from the diet—or when glucose can't get into cells, as in advanced diabetes—ketones build up to toxic levels. At first your breath has a weird odor, like fruit-flavored paint thinner. But soon you become confused, short of breath, and nauseous. You feel dehydrated and lose your lunch. If you don't get medical attention ASAP, you slip into a coma from which you may never awaken.

Since you're taking care of your diabetes, you'll likely never have to worry about

## Type 1 Diabetes: What Are the Odds?

| A baby born . . . | has the following risk for type 1 diabetes |
|---|---|
| To parents who do not have type 1 diabetes | 1 in 300 |
| To a mother 25 or older who has type 1 diabetes | 1 in 100* |
| To a mother younger than 25 who has type 1 diabetes | 1 in 25* |
| To a father who has type 1 diabetes | 1 in 17* |
| To a mother and father who have type 1 diabetes | Between 1 in 10 and 1 in 4 |
| With an identical twin who has type 1 diabetes | Between 1 in 4 and 1 in 2 |

*If the parent developed type 1 diabetes before age 11, the risk is doubled.*

this condition, called ketoacidosis. However, monitoring ketones is part of managing diabetes, which you'll learn about later in his chapter.

# Type 2 Diabetes

When your doctor uttered the words "You have type 2 diabetes," you were inducted into a fast-growing, nonexclusive club—a club no one wants to join. Some 90-95 percent of all people with diabetes in the United States have type 2. That adds up to more than 23 million Americans.

As was the case with type 1 diabetes, this condition used to go by other names, including non-insulin-dependent diabetes and adult-onset diabetes. Now it's clear that both terms are misnomers. More than one-third of people with type 2 diabetes require insulin injections, so a person with type 2 diabetes may indeed be insulin dependent. And type 2 isn't limited to adults, either. While most people who develop type 2 diabetes are

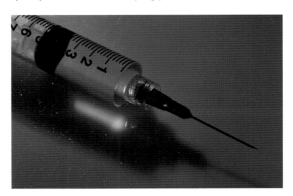

over 35, more and more kids are turning up in doctors' offices with classic type 2 diabetes, largely because more and more kids today are obese. As you read on, you'll learn why lugging around extra weight increases the risk for type 2 diabetes.

Unlike type 1 diabetes, type 2 diabetes is not an autoimmune disease, in which the body attacks its own cells. Type 2 typically begins with a phenomenon called insulin resistance, when cells throughout your body start to ignore insulin. The hormone comes knocking, but the doormen have trouble letting it in. The insulin may not be able to open the cell doors, or it may take reinforcements in the form of extra-large gushes of insulin before the cells will open up. In either case, glucose builds up in the blood.

Insulin resistance causes no symptoms. It's not as though you can feel or hear glucose molecules crashing into your resistant, tightly closed cells. However, insulin resistance often sets the stage for type 2 diabetes. Bottom line: If you have type 2 diabetes, you almost certainly have insulin resistance.

It usually takes insulin resistance months or years to progress to type 2 diabetes, when beta cells become progressively incapable of meeting the demand for insulin. At that point, insulin levels in the blood rise, too, as the beta cells keep cranking out the hormone in an attempt to coax open stubborn cells.

People often dismiss the signs and symptoms or blame them on some other health problem. A few indicators of type 2 diabetes overlap with those experienced by people with type 1, including:

- constant thirst
- frequent need to urinate
- increased hunger
- fatigue

However, type 2 diabetes often produces additional symptoms, such as:

- cuts that take a long time to heal
- frequent infections
- blurry eyesight
- tingling or numbness in the hands and feet
- erectile dysfunction

In all likelihood, your body began to experience insulin resistance long before you were diagnosed with type 2 diabetes, especially if you have any of the latter five symptoms. Excess glucose in the blood interferes with the work of white blood cells, which explains why cuts and sores take longer to heal. Meanwhile, germs snack on glucose, which makes them stronger, promoting more infections. Long-term exposure to glucose damages nerves, too, which explains many other symptoms that occur with type 2 diabetes.

While you may be able to live with these problems, they should serve as a loud, clear warning that your out-of-control blood sugar is slowly trashing your body like a rowdy rock band wrecks a hotel room. Left untreated, type 2 diabetes—or any type of diabetes, for that matter—can lead to medical catastrophe. You'll learn more about the potential damage in the next chapter.

## Gestational Diabetes

You're stuck wearing maternity clothes. You miss having a glass of wine with dinner. You can't see your feet when you stand up. And now you find out that your pregnancy is causing diabetes? Talk about frustrating. But at least you're not alone.

Gestational diabetes was thought to affect anywhere from 2 to 10 percent of pregnancies, but recent revisions in the way it is diagnosed may put that number as high as 18 percent. The condition usually doesn't arise until after 20 weeks of pregnancy. And while any pregnant woman can develop gestational diabetes, it's definitely more common if you:

- are older than 25
- have a parent or sibling with diabetes

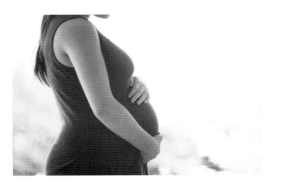

- are African American, American Indian, Asian American, Hispanic American, or Pacific Islander
- are overweight
- developed gestational diabetes during a previous pregnancy or have given birth to an infant who weighed more than nine pounds
- have ever been told by a doctor that you have prediabetes, impaired glucose tolerance, or impaired fasting glucose. (You'll read more about these conditions later in the chapter.)

So what's the harm in having high blood sugar for a few months? For starters, women with gestational diabetes often develop high blood pressure (referred to as pre-eclampsia), which brings its own risks for both mother and baby. What's more, they frequently give birth to very large babies who weigh more than nine pounds. Not only do fat babies often require a caesarean-section delivery, but they're also more likely to be fat children and to develop diabetes by their

teen years or young adulthood (because of their genetic inheritance, not the intrauterine environment).

The news about gestational diabetes isn't all bad. After all, there's a reliable cure for the problem: having your baby, after which most women's blood sugar levels return to normal.

However, the condition lingers in a small number of women, who are then diagnosed with either type 1 or type 2 diabetes. Regardless, if you have gestational diabetes once, the odds are two out of three that you'll develop it again with a subsequent pregnancy. More concerning, women who have gestational diabetes stand a 20 to 50 percent risk of developing type 2 diabetes within a decade.

## Other Types of Diabetes

Type 1, type 2, and gestational diabetes are the main types of the disease, but they're not the only ones. The following are other diabetes permutations.

## "Double" Diabetes

Although it's not a term you will find in most medical textbooks, many doctors today say they are treating a growing number of type 1 diabetes patients who have also developed insulin resistance, the classic symptom of type 2 diabetes. Some doctors are treating these hybrid patients with drugs that make their bodies more sensitive to insulin. The term "double diabetes" may also be used to describe a person with type 2 diabetes who develops antibodies that destroy the pancreatic beta cells (the ones that produce insulin); in most cases, these patients will require insulin injections. Just to make matters more confusing, double diabetes is sometimes called type 3 diabetes.

## Prediabetes

Think of it as "diabetes lite" or the diabetic gray zone. You have insulin resistance, so your blood sugar is higher than it should be, but it's not high enough for you to be diagnosed with type 2 diabetes. (We'll explain the values doctors use to measure blood sugar later in this chapter.) It has been estimated that about 35 percent of U.S. adults aged 20 and older (and 50 percent of those aged 65 and older) have prediabetes. Using the U.S. population in 2010, that means at least 79 million Americans aged 20 and older have prediabetes. Most people who have the condition develop full-blown type 2 diabetes within 10 years. However, making certain changes, such as losing weight, can delay or even prevent that from happening.

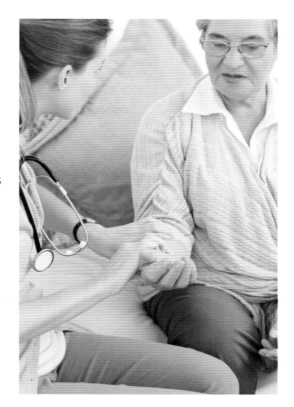

## Latent Autoimmune Diabetes of Adulthood (LADA)

LADA is also known as slow-onset type 1 diabetes. Call them late bloomers: About 5 to 10 percent of people with diabetes are adults who develop the type 1 variety of the condition, which is typically first diagnosed in children and teens. Doctors often mistake the condition for plain old type 2 diabetes, basing their diagnosis solely on a patient's age and high blood sugar. But people with LADA don't have

# Insulin and Your Heart

The oldest rule in the book is that too much of a good thing can make you sick, and that rule applies to insulin in a big way. While you need insulin to survive, sending gushers of the hormone into your blood can eventually damage arteries, which makes insulin resistance a cause of heart disease.

Insulin resistance is one part of a spectrum of conditions that make up the medical threat originally known as Syndrome X but now more commonly called metabolic syndrome or insulin resistance syndrome. The National Cholesterol Education Program defines metabolic syndrome as the presence of any three of the following conditions:

- Excess weight around the waist (that is, a waist measurement of more than 40 inches for men and more than 35 inches for women)
- High levels of blood fats called triglycerides (150 mg/dl or higher)
- Low levels of HDL ("good") cholesterol (below 40 mg/dl for men and below 50 mg/dl for women)
- High blood pressure (130/85 or higher)
- High fasting blood glucose levels (110 mg/dl or higher)

Other medical organizations use slightly different criteria for defining metabolic syndrome. And some doctors don't think metabolic syndrome exists at all, since it has no single cause; in addition to the cluster of factors mentioned above, other culprits include high levels of inflammation in the blood vessels and disorders that damage the endothelium, or lining of blood vessels. In fact, in recent years scientists have debated whether there's any point in using metabolic syndrome as a medical diagnosis. However, there is little argument about the fact that insulin resistance—the hallmark of type 2 diabetes—raises the risk of heart disease.

insulin resistance and aren't necessarily overweight. Those are important distinctions, since they influence which treatments work for LADA.

## Maturity-Onset Diabetes of the Young (MODY)

MODY is something like the flipside of LADA. It usually turns up in teens and young adults, although it may be found in children as well as older adults. Because patients tend to be youngish and slender, doctors often misdiagnose the condition as type 1 diabetes. However, MODY is a genetic disorder that interferes with insulin production. And unlike people with type 2 diabetes, those with MODY don't have insulin resistance. Again, getting the right diagnosis is critical in order to choose the proper treatment approach for MODY.

## Secondary Diabetes

Certain diseases and drug therapies pack a diabetic double whammy by making people more vulnerable to blood sugar problems, either by directly interfering with insulin or by producing physical changes that increase insulin resistance (such as weight gain) and can lead to diabetes. When another identifiable medical problem or medication precipitates the development of diabetes, it is called secondary diabetes. A brief list of conditions that may cause secondary diabetes includes depression, HIV, pancreatitis, certain hormonal disorders (such as Cushing's syndrome and hyperthyroidism), and some genetic disorders (such as cystic fibrosis). Drugs linked to secondary diabetes include diuretics and other drugs used to treat high blood pressure, steroid hormones, certain asthma medications, antidepressants, anticonvulsants, and some forms of cancer chemotherapy, among others.

## What Causes Diabetes?

Ask a doctor this question and you may get a long, complicated answer that leaves you wishing you hadn't opened your big mouth. Or you may get a shrug and this unsatisfying response: "Nobody knows."

In a sense, both answers are accurate. Scientists have pinpointed a number of genes that seem to be involved in creating your body's blood sugar problems. Yet they also know that one or more triggers in the environment are probably necessary, too. But what are those potential triggers? And how do they keep insulin from doing its job?

Researchers are still sorting out these questions, but in the following pages we'll take a look at what they know so far.

19

# Type 1 Diabetes

Some people inherit their mother's freckles or father's nose. If you have type 1 diabetes, there's a good chance one of your parents passed along to you an abnormal gene or cluster of genes that puts you at greater-than-average risk for developing the condition. (For those of you who were busy dozing or passing notes during high school biology class, everyone inherits a blend of genes from both parents that not only determines what you look like but also greatly influences your health.)

Being born with these genes doesn't guarantee that you will develop type 1 diabetes, however. These inherited genes only make you *susceptible* to developing diabetes. Something else has to trigger changes in your body to create your blood sugar problem. But what?

Scientists aren't sure, but they have a short list of suspects. According to one theory, a virus or some environmental toxin worms its way into the body and confuses the immune system because it resembles proteins found on beta cells. The immune system tends to shoot first and ask questions later, so it destroys anything

that looks like it could be a threat—including insulin-producing beta cells in the pancreas. Type 1 diabetes occurs more often in people who have had a viral illness, as this can trigger the onset of type 1 diabetes in a susceptible individual.

Other scientists have speculated that switching a baby from breast milk to cow's milk too early is the culprit. However, the dairy-diabetes connection remains controversial. In fact, in 2003 a pair of studies in the *Journal of the American Medical Association* found no connection between consuming cow's milk and diabetes.

Some causes are more clear-cut. For example, certain prescription medications can trigger type 1 diabetes (see Secondary Diabetes on page 19.)

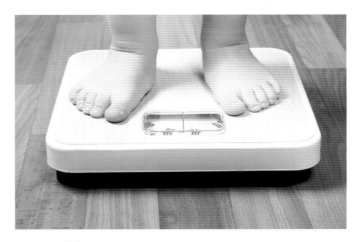

20

# Type 2 Diabetes

If you have type 2 diabetes, you may have begun to regret every can of cola and candy bar you ever consumed. After all, if high blood glucose is your problem, didn't gobbling and guzzling all that sugar cause you to develop diabetes?

The precise answer to that question is "Not exactly," though having a sweet tooth probably didn't help matters. Despite the common misconception, consuming sugary foods doesn't cause diabetes. However, eating too much of most any kind of food—whether it's bonbons or bacon cheeseburgers—can make you gain weight. And getting fat worsens insulin resistance, the problem that's at the core of type 2 diabetes.

Insulin resistance is the medical term for the concept described earlier: Cells throughout your body have begun to ignore insulin, so your pancreas keeps cranking out more of the hormone to move glucose past those stubborn cell membranes.

What causes insulin resistance? Typically, it is a combination of genetics (heredity) and lifestyle. Family history plays a major role. Having close relatives with type 2 diabetes greatly increases your risk of the disease. Certain ethnic groups, including

## Carrying a Heavy Burden

Currently, more than 78 million American adults are considered obese. Compared to adults who weigh a healthy amount, obese individuals are more than *seven times* as likely to develop diabetes. And the problem is not restricted to adults. An estimated 12.5 million kids in America today fall in the obese category. More than ever before, overweight children and teenagers are developing insulin resistance and type 2 diabetes.

Native Americans, African Americans, Hispanic Americans, Asian Americans, and Pacific Islanders are also at high risk. The aging process plays a role, too. The older we get, the more insulin resistant we tend to become, so the risk of developing type 2 diabetes increases with age.

Women who have a condition called polycystic ovary syndrome (PCOS) often become insulin resistant due to the overproduction of certain hormones that work against insulin's action.

Likewise, several hormones produced during pregnancy fight against insulin's action and can cause insulin resistance.

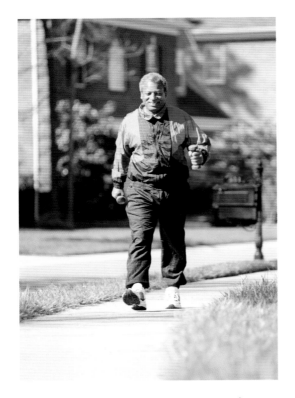

trigger this energy burst by stimulating the liver to release extra sugar into the bloodstream and by causing insulin resistance.

A number of medications can also produce insulin resistance, most notably, anti-inflammatory steroid drugs such as cortisone and prednisone. (See Secondary Diabetes on page 19.) These types of drugs create a state of insulin resistance throughout the body.

A lack of physical activity can cause insulin resistance in many people. The muscles are one of the primary consumers of sugar for energy. When muscle function is limited to little more than getting up to find the remote or to head to the fridge, muscles start to lose their sensitivity to insulin. Even in people who are usually very active, a couple of days without much activity will result in some degree of insulin resistance.

And as we noted earlier, women who develop gestational diabetes during pregnancy or have given birth to a large or heavy baby are at increased risk of developing type 2 diabetes as they get older.

Stressful circumstances, such as illness, injury, surgery, or daily emotional turmoil, can cause significant insulin resistance. This is due to the production of stress hormones. These hormones normally prompt the surge of energy needed for a "fight or flight" response in stressful situations. Unfortunately for people prone to diabetes, the stress hormones

Last but certainly not least, insulin resistance increases with body size. But let's get the terminology straight. We're not talking about being big and muscular. We're talking about having too much body fat, particularly around the midsection. Obesity (being more than 20 percent over one's ideal weight due to excess body fat) is far and away the number one risk factor for type 2

If you've been diagnosed with prediabetes, take it every bit as seriously as you would the full-fledged disease. Prediabetes means that you are already insulin resistant and that your pancreas is beginning to show signs of wear. You can bet your bottom dollar that, if you don't make some important lifestyle changes, your condition will progress to a more severe state. So attack diabetes early—before your pancreas loses its capabilities and resilience.

diabetes. We don't know exactly how body fat gets in the way of insulin. But we do know that fat cells secrete a hormone that limits insulin's ability to promote sugar uptake by the body's cells. The larger your fat cells, the more of this hormone you produce, and the greater your degree of insulin resistance. In fact, gaining as little as ten pounds over a 15-year period can double your level of insulin resistance.

Still, if some 79 million Americans have insulin resistance, how come less than half of them have developed type 2 diabetes? Why the discrepancy? The reason is this: When insulin resistance occurs, the pancreas needs to produce more insulin to keep blood sugar levels in a normal range. In most cases, the pancreas can produce enough extra insulin to keep

blood sugar levels out of the diabetic range, even though the insulin is not working as well as it should. This is the prediabetes phase.

But not everyone's pancreas has this capacity. Each person's pancreas can only crank up insulin production so much. Once the degree of insulin resistance is too much for the pancreas to overcome, blood sugar levels rise above normal. A body must have both insulin resistance *and* a limit to its ability to secrete extra insulin for type 2 diabetes to occur.

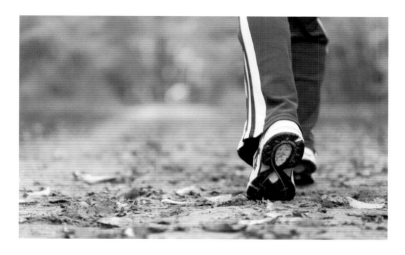

## No Coincidence

In a Gallup-Healthways survey conducted in 2012, six of the ten states with the highest obesity rates were also among the ten states with the highest rates of diabetes. Those states were (in alphabetical order): Alabama, Kentucky, Louisiana, Mississippi, Tennessee, and West Virginia.

To understand this concept better, imagine that you are an air conditioner trying to keep the house cool on a hot summer day. If you're one of those high-powered central air-conditioning units that can crank out a bazillion BTUs, you'll have no problem overcoming the heat and keeping the house cool. But if you're one of those inexpensive window units, you're probably not going to be able to blow enough cold air to keep the entire house cool on a really hot, humid day.

In this example, the heat and humidity are like insulin resistance: They present a challenge to our comfort and well-being. The air conditioner is like the pancreas: An efficient system can overcome any challenge, but a less-resilient system can't. When a sluggish pancreas combines with major insulin resistance, the result is going to be type 2 diabetes. Fortunately, at this early stage of type 2 diabetes, blood sugar control can often be achieved through exercise and a healthy diet. Physical activity, as we will discuss in a later chapter, helps the body overcome insulin resistance. Consuming fewer carbohydrates helps to limit the amount of sugar entering the bloodstream at any one time. And the combination of exercise and reduced food intake produces weight loss, which also improves insulin sensitivity. Sometimes at this stage, however, oral medications may also be needed to help the pancreas (or to help insulin) work more effectively. Combined with the lifestyle adjustments, they may be sufficient to rein in blood sugar levels, at least for a while.

However, type 2 diabetes is a progressive illness. The word *progressive* in this context does *not* mean something positive. There is nothing hip, cool, or modern about it. In this case, *progressive* means that the disease will grow worse and become harder to control over time. When diabetes has been present for a number of years, insulin resistance tends to grow worse, and the pancreas struggles to keep up with the huge demand for insulin. Then a new problem typically sets in. Just like an air conditioner that is forced to run full blast every minute of every day, the pancreas starts to break down. (Heck, if you were asked to work day after day without any breaks and with no end in sight, you would break down too...or at least find a new job!)

The breakdown of the pancreas has two causes: Overwork and a condition known as glucose toxicity. The overwork part, we can all understand: Force those poor little pancreatic cells into relentless labor, and many of them are going to bite the dust. But glucose toxicity is a bit more complex. Glucose is a good thing in the right amounts. But elevations in blood sugar levels can actually damage the pancreas, further reducing its ability to produce insulin. So over time, as a result of the constant battle against insulin resistance, the pancreas starts to make less and less insulin. This is why the treatment for type 2 diabetes usually must become more aggressive over time. It is why

roughly 40 percent of the people with type 2 diabetes take insulin injections, sometimes several times each day. Does this mean they now have type 1 diabetes? No, it does not. Remember, the type of diabetes is defined by what *caused* it, not how it is treated. Type 1 diabetes occurs when the body's own immune system destroys the part of the pancreas that makes insulin. Type 2 diabetes is caused by insulin resistance (usually due to obesity and family history/ ethnicity), followed by insufficient insulin production (as the pancreas fails to keep up with the increased demand), followed by a gradual breakdown of the pancreas (due to constant overwork and glucose toxicity).

## How Does My Doctor Know I Have Diabetes?

Your blood sugar gives you away, of course. Doctors do look for other clues when considering a diagnosis of diabetes—outward symptoms, for example, or the presence of risk factors, such as overweight or a family history of the disease. But a firm diagnosis of diabetes isn't made until the blood is tested.

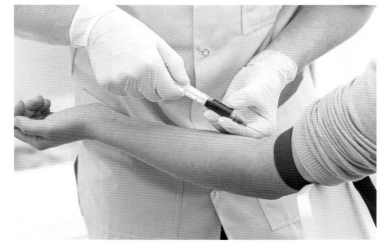

If a patient walks in complaining that he or she is unusually thirsty and always dashing for the restroom, for instance, a physician may suspect diabetes, especially the type 1 variety. But the diagnosis can't be confirmed until the blood sugar level is tested. For a patient exhibiting symptoms that are common with diabetes, a doctor may order a *random blood glucose (RBG)* test. This test can be performed at any time and doesn't require preparation. A result that shows a blood sugar level more than 200 milligrams per deciliter (mg/dl) suggests diabetes is present.

Since prediabetes and the early stages of type 2 diabetes often don't cause outward symptoms, however, a doctor may order a blood test called an *HbA1c,* often shortened to *A1c,* to check for diabetes in a patient who is over age 45 (the risk of type 2 diabetes increases with age), is overweight, or has any other risk factor for the disease. At one time, A1c testing (explained in greater detail in Chapter 4) was used only as a method for evaluating diabetes management. But in 2009 an international committee of diabetes experts determined that the test could also be used in most cases for diagnosing prediabetes and type 2 diabetes. Like an RBG test, an A1c test can be performed at any time of day and doesn't require fasting beforehand. The A1c results reflect a patient's average blood glucose level over the previous two to three months. An A1c of 5.7 to 6.4 indicates prediabetes; a level of 6.5 or

## Are You Overweight?

Stepping on the scale doesn't tell the whole story. Doctors use body mass index (BMI) to determine whether a person's weight is proportionate to their height. If your BMI falls between 25 and 29, you're overweight. If it's 30 or higher, you are considered obese.

Here's how to calculate your BMI:

1) Weigh yourself first thing in the morning, without clothes.
2) Confirm your height, in inches.
3) Multiply your weight in pounds by 700.
4) Divide the result in step 3 by your height in inches.
5) Divide the result in step 4 by your height in inches again.

The resulting number is your BMI.

| Blood Glucose: What the Tests Tell | | | |
|---|---|---|---|
| | HbA1c (percent) | FPG (mg/dL) | OGTT (mg/dL) |
| Diabetes | 6.5 or higher | 126 or higher | 200 or higher |
| Prediabetes | 5.7 to 6.4 | 100 to 125 | 140 to 199 |
| Normal | Below 5.7 | 99 or lower | 139 or lower |

above means the patient has diabetes. Another option for diagnosing prediabetes and diabetes is a *fasting plasma glucose (FPG)* test. This test is more definitive than an RBG test and is often included in the routine blood analyses conducted as part of annual physical examinations. Before 2009, it was the most common test used for diagnosing diabetes and is still relied upon by many doctors and health care facilities.

If you have had an FPG test, you probably haven't forgotten it, especially if you love breakfast. As the name implies, the test measures how much blood sugar is in your system when your stomach is empty.

Everyone's glucose spikes after eating a meal, but sugar levels drop within a few hours in people who do not have diabetes. In those with diabetes, blood sugar remains relatively high long after the dishes have been cleared and washed.

If an FPG test is ordered, the patient typically receives instructions not to eat after midnight on the day before the test and then to arrive at a lab bright and early to provide a blood sample. After the blood has been drawn, as the hungry patient bolts for the nearest coffee shop, the lab analyzes the blood. If the test produces a reading lower than 100 mg/dl, diabetes is not present. A reading of 126 mg/dl or higher is a red flag, but

## One Reason to Be a Morning Person?

Having a fasting plasma glucose test performed in the morning may help you get a proper diagnosis. The reason? Doctors diagnose diabetes when a patient's blood sugar level measures 126 mg/dl or higher on two consecutive FPG tests. Scientists established the threshold of 126 mg/dl based on studies of blood sugar levels measured in the morning after an eight-hour fast. But sometimes patients undergo an FPG test in the afternoon. That's a problem, because many people—including all people with diabetes—experience a spike in blood sugar, known as the "dawn phenomenon," between 4 a.m. and 8 a.m. Blood sugar naturally dips by afternoon. A study in 2000 compared two groups of more than 6,000 people who underwent blood-sugar testing. One group went to the lab in the morning, the other in the afternoon. The study found that people tested in the morning were twice as likely to be diagnosed with diabetes. Since people in both groups were similar ages and had comparable health status, the researchers estimated that using current standards for blood-sugar testing in the afternoon may miss up to half of all cases of undiagnosed diabetes.

since other influences, such as stress and certain illnesses, can raise blood sugar, doctors usually order a retest to confirm the diagnosis.

Inquiring minds may wonder: What if an FPG result is above 100 mg/dl but below 126 mg/dl? If that's the case, the patient has a form of prediabetes called *impaired fasting glucose*. In short, it means the patient doesn't yet have diabetes but may join the club one day one day. A reading in this middle zone offers a strong clue that insulin resistance has been present for some time.

If any of these tests indicates that a patient's blood sugar is close to normal but the doctor has some reason to suspect diabetes (for instance, if the patient has classic symptoms of the condition), another kind of test may be ordered to clarify matters. An *oral glucose tolerance test (OGTT)* measures how well the body processes sugar that surges into the bloodstream after a meal.

This test is more sensitive than the FBG test, since it does a better job of detecting prediabetes. However, the OGTT takes longer to perform and involves more hassle for the patient. As with the FBG test, it requires that the patient consume nothing but water for eight hours prior to testing. After the patient's blood sugar is measured once, he or she is given a drink containing 75 grams of glucose. Two hours later, a lab technician measures the blood sugar a second time. A result of 139 mg/dl or lower means the patient does not have diabetes. A blood sugar level between 140 and 199 mg/dl is called *impaired glucose tolerance*, a second type of prediabetes. If the reading is 200 mg/dl or higher, the patient is told to come back for a repeat test. A second result above 200 mg/dl indicates diabetes is present.

Other tests may be performed to determine the type of diabetes present. High levels of islet-cell antibodies in the blood, low levels of a substance called C-peptide in the blood (which indicates how much insulin the body is making), and high levels of ketones in the urine all indicate type 1 diabetes.

A diagnosis can be scary. However, once you have a diagnosis, you can take steps to put yourself in control of the disease.

# Get Motivated

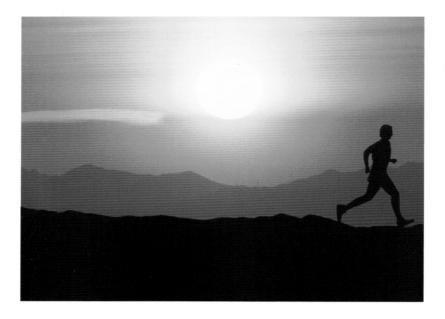

Managing diabetes takes commitment and effort on your part. There's no two ways about it. So it's understandable that you might wonder what's really in it for you. Why should you bother putting in the time and energy to get and keep your blood sugar levels under control?

There may be no better motivation for stabilizing your blood sugar than the fear of living with—or dying from—the devastating long-term complications that are likely to occur if you don't. In this chapter, we give you a glimpse at those potential complications—not only to educate you but to give you real incentive to walk the path of control. And in case the prospect of a bleak future isn't enough to light your diabetes-fighting fire, we also reveal some of the immediate, tangible improvements that can come from reining in your blood sugar.

# Think of Your Future

Perhaps you know or have heard of someone who wound up going blind, losing a foot, or needing kidney dialysis as a result of diabetes. Unfortunately, that's only the tip of the iceberg when it comes to the long-term effects of poorly controlled diabetes. Diabetes can produce a number of serious consequences if you don't take good care of yourself and manage your condition properly.

If the thought of your body decaying and falling apart strikes serious fear into you, *good!* Fear can be a powerful motivator. It's what keeps us from doing stupid things like playing with fire and picking fights with people twice our size. And maybe, just maybe, it will inspire you to control your blood sugar. Some of the proven long-term benefits of quality blood sugar management include:

- improved heart health
- better blood flow
- healthy kidneys
- proper nerve function
- less nerve pain
- fit feet
- clear vision
- mental soundness
- healthy teeth and gums
- flexible joints
- a positive outlook

# Improved Heart Health

Despite the long list of health problems diabetes can cause, heart disease is what ultimately kills the majority of people with diabetes. People with diabetes are at least twice as likely to develop heart disease and two to four times more likely to die from it than are people without diabetes. Why? To begin with, many people with diabetes are overweight and have elevated blood cholesterol and blood pressure levels, any one of which on its own increases the risk of heart disease. But diabetes itself is considered a major risk factor for heart disease because having excess sugar in the bloodstream threatens the heart. Sugar is a sticky substance (think of the last time you ate cotton candy or spilled juice). It makes cholesterol, fat, and other substances in the blood stick to the interior walls of blood vessels, contributing to the formation of plaque. Plaque makes blood vessels thick and inflexible, a condition

## Heart Health

In addition to having an increased risk of developing and dying from heart disease, people with diabetes also tend to develop heart trouble at an earlier age than do folks without diabetes.

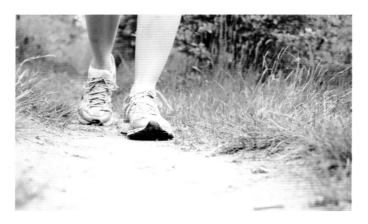

other vital body parts require large amounts of oxygen and depend on healthy blood vessels to deliver an unobstructed flow of oxygen-rich blood. The most important of these is the brain. When a blood vessel leading to the brain becomes clogged with sticky plaque, the brain cells normally fed by that vessel do not receive enough oxygen and quickly die. This is called a stroke. The risk of stroke is two to four times higher for people who have diabetes than in people who do not have it.

The muscles in the legs also depend on a reliable and substantial flow of blood. When blood vessels that feed the legs become clogged, the leg muscles don't get sufficient oxygen, which can lead to pain or cramping during exercising or walking. This condition is called claudication. Blood vessel disease in the legs is *20 times* more common in people with diabetes than in those without it. Claudication occurs in 15 percent of people who have had diabetes for 10 years and 45 percent of those who have had it for 20 years.

known as atherosclerosis, or hardening of the arteries. The thickening of the blood vessel walls narrows the space through which the blood flows, slowing its passage. And sometimes pieces of plaque break off, which may lead to the formation of blood clots that further restrict the flow of blood to vital organs such as the heart.

**The good news:** Improving blood sugar control dramatically reduces the risk of heart disease. In addition to preventing the formation of much of the plaque that clogs blood vessels, better diabetes management also frequently leads to reductions in blood cholesterol and blood pressure levels. Plus, the positive lifestyle steps you take to control blood sugar, such as exercising regularly, eating more healthfully, and cutting back on stress, further reduce your risk of heart disease.

## Better Blood Flow

In addition to the heart, a number of

**The good news:** Tightening blood sugar control, along with all the other changes and lifestyle improvements that come with it, will help blood flow more freely to all the vital body parts. For people with diabetes who have already developed circulatory problems, symptoms often decrease as blood sugar levels improve.

## Healthy Kidneys

Visit any kidney dialysis center and check the charts of the people who sit there for hours a day, several days a week, with tubes in their arms, hooked up to machines that filter waste products, toxins, and other undesirable substances from their blood. Diabetic. Diabetic. Not diabetic. Diabetic. Diabetic. Get the idea?

Diabetes is the leading cause of kidney failure, accounting for 44 percent of new cases of kidney disease. More than 200,000 Americans with diabetes have received kidney transplants or are receiving dialysis treatment.

### Losing Their Edge

Women who have not yet experienced menopause have a far lower risk for heart disease than men do, possibly as a result of the beneficial effects of hormones. However, having diabetes erases the hormones' protective effects: Women with diabetes have the same risk for heart disease as men, regardless of their age.

Approximately 50,000 Americans with diabetes begin treatment for end-stage renal (kidney) disease each year. Minorities, especially African Americans and Hispanics, who have type 2 diabetes are highly susceptible to kidney disease, but everyone with elevated blood sugar levels is at risk. Elevated blood sugar damages the tiny blood vessels, called capillaries, that form and nourish the filters within the kidneys.

**The good news:** Tightening blood sugar control dramatically reduces the risk of kidney disease. In fact, major studies examining the effect of blood sugar levels on kidney disease found that every 30 mg/dl drop in average blood sugar leads to a 30 percent reduction in the risk of kidney disease.

## Proper Nerve Function

The nervous system is like the body's electrical wiring, relaying signals that control voluntary and involuntary functions throughout the body. A portion of that interior wiring, called the autonomic nervous system, controls the body's involuntary activities. Those activities include all of the basic, "behind the scenes" functions—such as the beating of the heart, the digestion of food, the regulation of body temperature, the maintenance of balance, and the physical response to sexual stimulation—

## Damage Control

Autonomic neuropathy is difficult to treat, but controlling your blood sugar levels can prevent or delay the onset of these troublesome symptoms. In a major study on the complications of diabetes, patients who maintained tight control of their glucose levels reduced their risk for autonomic nerve damage by more than 50 percent.

that occur without conscious thought or direction on our part.

Nerves are like any other living tissue in the body: They use sugar for energy, and they require an unobstructed blood supply to provide them with oxygen and other nutrients. Excess sugar in the blood appears to cause two main problems for the nervous system. First, it interferes with the blood supply to the nerves—just as it interferes with the flow of blood to other parts of the body—by contributing to plaque buildup in the blood vessel walls. Second, high blood sugar seems to alter energy metabolism (the process of using sugar to fuel cell functions) in such a way that the nerves swell and the coating on the outside of the nerve fibers fails to do its job of insulating and protecting the nerves. When the nerves that regulate basic body functions are damaged in

this way by high blood sugar levels, the condition is referred to as autonomic neuropathy.

Population-based studies have shown that 60 to 70 percent of people with diabetes have some form of mild to severe nerve damage. For example, nearly 50 percent of all men with diabetes develop impotency within a decade of diagnosis, due mainly to malfunction of the nerves that produce an erection. Men who suffer from diabetes also tend to develop problems with erectile dysfunction as much as 10 to 15 years earlier than men who don't have diabetes. Women with diabetes are more likely than women without it to suffer from vaginal dryness, again as a result of damage to nerves that control sexual response. One study found that 18 percent of women with type 1 diabetes and 42 percent of those with type 2 experienced sexual dysfunction.

Nerve damage can also lead to delayed digestion, a condition known as gastroparesis that affects an estimated 25 to 55 percent of people with diabetes (30 percent of those with type 2), especially those who spent many years with uncontrolled blood sugar. Gastroparesis can cause painful bloating and, because it delays the peaking of blood sugar that normally occurs after a meal, can make diabetes even harder to control.

Postural hypotension, yet another condition caused by damage to nerves, is twice as common in people with diabetes. It is a type of low blood pressure that occurs during abrupt changes in position, such as standing up quickly from a seated or prone position, and can lead to dizziness and fainting.

**The good news:** Blood sugar control is an effective means of preventing all forms of autonomic neuropathy. And while autonomic neuropathy is not always reversible once it has developed, the condition may regress slightly or at least won't progress as quickly once blood sugar levels are returned to normal.

## Less Nerve Pain

As previously mentioned, 60 to 70 percent of all people with diabetes develop some form of nerve damage in their lifetime. Of those, most develop a form called peripheral neuropathy—malfunction of the nerves serving the limbs, especially the lower legs and feet. In its early stages, peripheral neuropathy expresses itself as tingling or numbness. But as it progresses and nerves become inflamed, it can cause constant and sometimes severe pain. While there are several conventional and alternative medical treatments for painful neuropathy, many sufferers find little or no relief.

## Good News!

Studies have shown that by dropping pounds and getting more active, people with prediabetes can delay or prevent type 2 diabetes and even return their blood sugar levels to the normal range.

**The good news:** Tight blood sugar control can help to minimize the pain and slow the progression of peripheral neuropathy. Even better, if it is initiated early enough in the course of diabetes, tight control may actually prevent peripheral neuropathy from developing in the first place.

## Fit Feet

Yet another problem resulting from peripheral neuropathy is the risk of serious foot infections and deformities. How can a nerve problem lead to infection? It's a rather simple chain reaction. If, because of numbness, you cannot feel a minor foot injury and so continue to use that foot, the injury can grow more severe. If there is inadequate blood flow to the injured area to aid in the healing process—a likely scenario considering the circulation problems common among people with diabetes—an infection can easily develop. As the infection spreads into the underlying tissue and bone, portions of the foot suffer cell death, a condition known as gangrene.

Foot deformities often develop because the nerves that coordinate complex movements in the feet fail to do their job. The person with neuropathy may put pressure on inappropriate (or injured) areas of the foot and cause further damage that goes unnoticed due to the lack of pain sensation.

Each year, roughly 70,000 Americans with diabetes require lower-limb amputations. Diabetes is the underlying reason for more amputations than all other causes combined, and loss of protective nerve sensation is the most critical factor. Even more disturbing is the fact that most people with diabetes who have a toe, foot, or limb amputated die within three years.

**The good news:** Tight blood sugar control helps to preserve sufficient blood flow to the feet. It helpls preserve healthy nerve function as well.

In addition, as you'll learn later in this chapter, lowering blood sugar levels helps to reduce the risk of infection in general. That's really good news for those looking to prevent foot problems as well as those recovering from existing foot ailments.

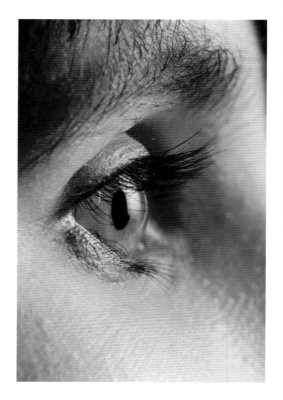

# Clear Vision

In the back of the eye is a sensitive layer of tissue called the retina that acts much like the film in a camera. The retina receives and records light from the outside world. Those images in light are then converted into electrical signals that are transmitted to the brain to produce vision. A network of capillaries provides the living cells of the retina with oxygen and nutrients. Elevated blood sugar levels, however, weaken these tiny blood vessels. As a result, they may swell, leak, or grow in unhealthy ways, blocking light from ever reaching the retina. This condition is called diabetic retinopathy.

Diabetes is the leading cause of new cases of blindness among adults ages 20 to 74. Diabetic retinopathy accounts for 12,000 to 20,000 new cases of blindness each year. In fact, roughly one of every five people with type 2 diabetes already has retinopathy when they are diagnosed with diabetes. Glaucoma, cataracts, and diseases of the cornea (the transparent outer covering of the eyeball) are also more common in people with diabetes and contribute to the high rate of blindness among this population.

**The good news:** Tight blood sugar control reduces the risk of retinopathy. Every 30 mg/dl reduction in average blood sugar lowers the risk of retinopathy by approximately 30 percent. For those with existing retinopathy, tightening blood sugar control slows the progression significantly.

# Mental Soundness

With aging comes increased risk for a number of health problems. Few instill as much fear as Alzheimer's disease, a progressive and ultimately fatal disease that destroys brain cells, causing increasingly severe problems with memory, thinking, and behavior along the way. Today, it affects more than five million Americans and is the sixth-leading cause of death in the United States. Currently, there is no cure for Alzheimer's. Damaged blood vessels in the brain are believed to play a role in the development of Alzheimer's. And recent research suggests that people with diabetes are more than twice as likely to develop Alzheimer's compared to those with normal glucose tolerance.

**The good news:** If you have type 2 diabetes, tight blood sugar control can reduce your risk of Alzheimer's disease to that of the general nondiabetic population.

# Healthy Teeth & Gums

Adults with diabetes have two times the risk of developing gum disease (periodontitis) as do their peers without diabetes. Almost one-third of people with diabetes have severe gum disease. Specifically, those with type 2 diabetes have greater plaque buildup and more bacteria below the gumline; as a result, their gums bleed more easily, and they commonly experience loosening and loss of teeth. Once a gum infection starts, it can take a long time to eradicate it when blood sugar is out of whack. Conversely, research has shown that having periodontal disease may make it more difficult for people who have diabetes to control their blood sugar levels.

**The good news:** Good blood sugar control can help prevent dental problems.

The lower the average blood sugar level, the lower the risk of gum disease and tooth loss.

## Flexible Joints

Joint mobility problems, including conditions such as frozen shoulder, trigger finger, and clawing of the hand, affect approximately 20 percent of people with diabetes, and high blood sugar is the root cause. Excess sugar in the blood sticks to collagen, a protein found in bone, cartilage, and tendons.

When collagen becomes sugar-coated, it thickens and stiffens, preventing joints from moving smoothly through their full range of motion and often causing joint pain.

**The good news:** Keeping your blood sugar levels near normal reduces your risk of developing joint mobility problems. And if you already have limited range of motion in your shoulders, hands, fingers, or other joints, lowering your blood sugar levels may help improve your range of motion and limit the pain associated with stiff joints.

## A Positive Outlook

Blood sugar levels have a direct effect on our mental well-being. It is common for people with diabetes to feel down when their blood sugar levels are up. Depression is three to four times more common in adults with diabetes than in the general population. The mechanism of this increased risk is not entirely known. Since depression is often biochemical in nature, elevated sugar levels in the brain may play a direct role. It could also be related, at least in part, to the extra stress associated with living with a chronic illness. Certainly, developing complications from diabetes can instill a feeling of helplessness, a definite contributing factor in the onset of depression.

**The good news:** Improving your blood sugar levels can make you a happier person. Researchers at Harvard Medical School and the Joslin Diabetes Center studied the effects of blood sugar control on mood and disposition. They found that people with lower blood sugar levels reported a higher overall quality of life. Significantly better ratings were given in the areas of physical, emotional, and general health and vitality.

# Focus on the Immediate Gains

The long-term effects of diabetes and the long-term benefits of improved blood sugar control may indeed help inspire you to start taking your disease more seriously. But what really tends to motivate most people is immediate gratification. So in the following pages we discuss some of the concrete ways in which you will be rewarded right away for getting your blood sugar levels under control, including:

- Increased energy
- More restful sleep
- Improved physical performance
- Decreased appetite
- Heightened brain power
- More stable moods and emotions
- Fewer sick days
- Softer skin and healthier gums
- Greater personal safety

To provide yourself with powerful reasons to begin managing your diabetes today, try focusing on the many impressive benefits that start coming your way as soon as you start corralling your runaway blood sugar levels.

# Increased Energy

Raise your hand if you like being tired all the time. Okay, raise your hand if you're too tired to raise your hand. Elevated blood sugar reduces your overall energy level. Remember, high blood sugar is a sign that not enough sugar is getting into your body's cells, where it is used for energy. The fuel is there; it's just stuck in the bloodstream, kind of like a fleet of gasoline trucks that drive around aimlessly instead of unloading at your local gas station. This shortage of fuel inside the body's cells causes sleepiness and sluggishness. Even if the blood sugar is only elevated temporarily, the lack of energy will be noticeable during that time. As soon as the blood sugar returns to normal, the energy level usually improves. So forget the gimmicky "energy drinks." If you want more energy, control your diabetes!

# More Restful Sleep

We all know how important a good night's sleep is to feeling well and being productive the following day. Unfortunately, diabetes makes you more

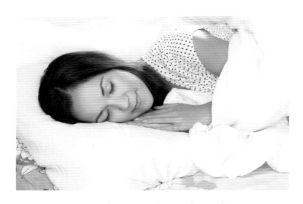

prone to developing sleep disorders, including sleep apnea, a potentially life-threatening disorder in which the sleeper snores loudly and actually stops breathing multiple times throughout the night. Poor blood sugar control also reduces the *quality* of your sleep. If you've ever woken up from a really long night's sleep feeling as though you hardly got any rest at all, it may be because you never reached a deep phase of sleep. Having elevated blood sugar during the night keeps you at a shallow sleep level and prevents you from entering the deep, restful sleep you really need.

If your blood sugar is high enough, you might even wake up several times during the night to run to the bathroom. This is caused by a condition called urine diuresis. When blood sugar reaches more than twice the normal level, some of the sugar spills into the urine, dragging a lot of water along with it. As the bladder fills, it wakes you up. The result may be frequent nighttime urination. If the thought of a restful, uninterrupted night's sleep appeals to you, start getting your blood sugar levels under control now

## Decreased Appetite

It might sound totally backward, but high blood sugar levels tend to make you crave

### Stay Vigilant

While maintaining tight control of blood sugar can greatly reduce the risk of developing serious health problems related to diabetes, there are no guarantees. So it's important to stay alert to the possible signs that a complication is developing. Early detection and treatment are key to minimizing the damage. At least once a year, see your ophthalmologist for an eye exam. Have your teeth cleaned and your gums checked for signs of periodontal disease at least twice, but preferably several times, a year. And have your feet examined and tested for adequate nerve sensation every time you visit your physician. (To remind yourself and your physician to perform this quick check, take off your shoes and socks once you're sitting in the exam room.) You'll find more information on fending off diabetes complications in Chapter 11: Protect and Prevent.

more food—especially carbohydrate-rich food. Remember, when it comes to appetite, it's not the amount of sugar in the bloodstream that counts, it's how much of that sugar gets into the body's cells. If not enough is getting into the cells, particularly the cells that regulate appetite, the body is going to feel hungry no matter how much food is eaten. Given that weight control is so important to both diabetes management and to your long-term health, it makes all the sense in the world to control your diabetes as best you can.

## Improved Physical Performance

Elevated blood sugar can reduce your strength, flexibility, speed, and stamina. So whether you're an aspiring athlete or just hoping to make it up a flight of stairs, you can immediately boost your physical abilities by gaining control of your blood sugar.

Muscles prefer sugar as fuel when they make quick, intense movements. When the sugar in the bloodstream can't get into the muscle cells, therefore, strength suffers. Extra sugar in the bloodstream also leads to something called glycosylation of connective tissues, in which sugar coats tendons and ligaments, limiting their ability to stretch properly. Muscle stiffness, strains, and pulls are common in people with high blood sugar levels. High blood sugar also gunks up the connections between muscles and nerves, resulting in dulled reflexes and slower reaction times. And extra sugar in the bloodstream limits the ability of red blood cells to pick up oxygen in the lungs and transport it to working muscles, causing rapid fatigue and restricted cardiovascular/aerobic capacity. So if you want to be able to perform well physically—during sports, exercise, or simple everyday activities—control your diabetes!

## Heightened Brain Power

Blood sugar levels influence more than your muscles, ligaments, and tendons, however. They affect your brain, too. High blood sugar limits your ability to focus, remember, perform complex tasks, and be creative. Studies have repeatedly and consistently shown that mental performance suffers during periods of high blood sugar. As blood sugar goes up, so do mental errors and the time it takes to perform basic tasks. Wide variations in blood sugar levels, from early-morning lows to postmeal spikes, have also been shown to hinder intellectual function. If you (or your loved ones) have noticed a decline in your mental abilities, tightening control of your diabetes might be the answer. Likewise, if you want to perform as well as you possibly can at work, in school, or in a friendly game of bridge, be vigilant about tracking and balancing those blood sugar levels.

## More Stable Moods & Emotions

Besides intellectual performance, your brain is also responsible for maintaining your emotional balance. The fact is, your moods change along with your blood sugar level. (If you don't believe it, ask your partner!) High blood sugar levels can make you impatient, irritable, and generally negative. Achieving normal blood sugar levels and keeping them there can go a long way toward improving your mood and your emotional stability. That's not to say that you will become an instant optimist or the life of the party. But the way you interact with your family, friends, coworkers, and even perfect strangers truly can impact your success and happiness in life. If you want to be on a more even keel, try evening out your blood sugar levels.

## Fewer Sick Days

Bacteria and viruses *love* sugar. They gobble it up and use it to grow and multiply. When blood sugar levels are up, the levels of sugar in virtually all of the body's tissues and fluids rise as well. That makes the diabetic body an ideal breeding ground for infection. If you ignore your high blood sugar levels, therefore, you are essentially supplying

## Which Came First?

Having diabetes can increase a person's risk of becoming depressed, but research published in 2010 suggests the reverse may also be true—that being depressed can increase one's odds of developing type 2 diabetes. The ten-year study looked at more than 65,000 women who were 50 to 75 years old in 1996. Participants who had diabetes at the start of the study turned out to be nearly 30 percent more likely to develop depression; for those who used insulin to control blood sugar, the likelihood of developing depression was over 50 percent. But in a bit of a twist, study subjects who were depressed actually had a 17 percent greater chance of developing type 2 diabetes over the course of the study—even after researchers made adjustments for diabetes risk factors such as inactivity and overweight, which also tend to be more common in people who are depressed. The researchers suggested that antidepressant medications as well as the body's own stress hormones—which can affect the body's ability to control blood sugar as well as the way it stores fat—may play some role in the increased diabetes risk.

## Sweet Job?

Diabetes mellitus, the disease's full scientific name, is actually Latin for "urine like honey." The fact that people with diabetes have high levels of sugar in their urine has been recognized for thousands of years. The ancient Greeks used to describe diabetes as a mysterious illness that involved the melting down of flesh and limbs into urine. In A.D. 300, Indian and Chinese scholars observed that the urine of people with diabetes was remarkably sweet. Indeed, in ancient times, diabetes was commonly diagnosed by "water tasters" who sampled the urine (referred to back then as "water") of those suspected of having diabetes in order to detect the telltale sweetness. Luckily for the water tasters, another method of sugar detection soon replaced this practice: The urine was poured near an anthill instead. If the ants were attracted to the urine, it meant that the urine contained high levels of sugar.

extra nutrients to the bad guys. Think of it as aiding and abetting the enemy. Everything from common colds and the flu to sinus infections and vaginal yeast infections are more common when blood sugar levels are elevated. And once illnesses and infections set in, they are much more difficult to shake when blood sugar is high. In fact, people with diabetes are much more likely to die from pneumonia or influenza than are people who do not have diabetes.

Research has shown that people who have better blood sugar control spend significantly fewer days absent from work, sick in bed, and restricted from their usual activities. So if you don't like—

or can't afford—to get sick, take better care of your diabetes!

## Softer Skin & Healthier Gums

Two other body parts that are affected immediately by changes in blood sugar levels are the skin and gums. The softness of your skin is greatly influenced by your level of hydration. When your blood sugar is high, your body tends to become dehydrated (due to urine diuresis, discussed previously). This leads to dry, cracked skin that can be more than uncomfortable and unsightly; it can open the door to infection, since the skin is your body's first line of defense against harmful bacteria and other microbes.

Maintaining your blood sugar near normal helps to prevent dehydration and keep your skin intact, soft, and supple.

Your gums are also immediately affected by changes in your blood sugar levels. Blood vessels bring oxygen-rich blood to the gum tissue to nourish it. However, if the blood has a high sugar content, that same blood flow can encourage the rapid growth of bacteria living below the gumline. After feasting on the sugar, the bacteria form plaque at an accelerated rate, contributing to bleeding gums and tooth loss. Controlling your diabetes will help reduce plaque buildup immediately and help you keep your natural teeth in your mouth, where they belong.

# Greater Personal Safety

Driving a car, operating machinery, crossing a street, and climbing stairs can all be dangerous, even deadly, undertakings for you and for those around you if you have uncontrolled blood sugar levels. You've already learned how high blood sugar (known in medical terms as hyperglycemia) can cause sleepiness and slow reaction times—a recipe for disaster when driving. But the opposite extreme, hypoglycemia, or low blood sugar, can be even more dangerous. It can put you in a coma and even kill you if it's not treated quickly enough.

Hypoglycemia can occur in anyone with diabetes who injects insulin or takes an oral diabetes medication that stimulates the pancreas to produce extra insulin, including a sulfonylurea (glipizide or glyburide) or a meglitinide (repaglinide or nateglinide).

A blood sugar level that is below normal usually causes the brain (as well as other body systems) to malfunction. Decision-making ability, judgment, and even awareness become impaired.

## Trumping Diabetes

U.S. Olympic swimmer Gary Hall Jr. was diagnosed with diabetes in 1999. At the time of his diagnosis, he had competed for, but had never won, an individual gold medal. Even his doctors doubted that he would ever win a coveted individual gold after he developed diabetes. But through an intensive insulin program that helped him achieve very tight control of his blood sugar, Gary proved everyone wrong, capturing the individual gold in the 50-meter freestyle at the 2000 Olympics and again at the 2004 Games.

Coordination suffers, and trembling can occur. So if you want to do all that you can to keep yourself and those around you safe, you must avoid blood sugar extremes by controlling your blood sugar levels. (You'll find more information on hyperglycemia and hypoglycemia in Chapter 10: Beware Highs and Lows.)

So as you've just discovered, almost every aspect of your physical and mental well-being is influenced by your blood sugar levels. Improving your blood sugar control will enable you to feel and perform better today and enjoy a healthier and more comfortable life for many tomorrows.

And that's some mighty powerful motivation to start (and continue) managing your diabetes. As you do, don't be afraid to ask for help!

# Enlist Help

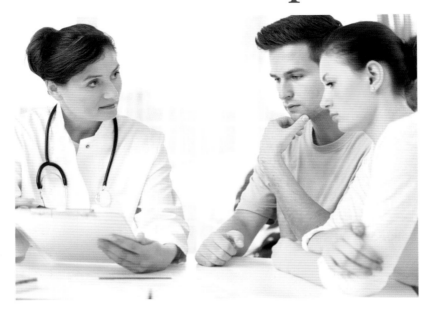

Now that you know a bit more about diabetes in general and why managing it properly is so important, you're probably anxious to start getting your condition under control. But where exactly do you begin, and what will you need to do to succeed?

To get the practical information, personalized advice, treatments, and support you need to begin successfully controlling your diabetes, you need to surround yourself with knowledgeable, experienced, trustworthy experts who can help you: In other words, you need to build your very own diabetes care team.

# Recruit Pros

If you haven't already, find a doctor who not only has skill and experience in diagnosing and treating diabetes but also one who will support and work with you in becoming the "boss" of your diabetes care. (Yes, that's right: Even though you are assembling a team of diabetes experts, you will ultimately remain responsible for your care. After all, *your* body and *your* future are on the line.) Together you and your doctor need to develop a good working relationship where there is mutual understanding, respect, and trust. You will need to feel comfortable talking honestly and openly with—and asking questions of—your doctor. If you are unable to develop such a relationship, you need to find another doctor.

Look for either an endocrinologist—a physician specially trained to treat people with hormone-related disorders such as diabetes—or an internist or general practitioner who has extensive experience in treating people with diabetes. You can get a list of the doctors in your area by contacting the American Diabetes Association (ADA) at 1-800-DIABETES or visiting their website at www.diabetes.org. If you cannot find a specialist near you, pick a primary care doctor who will work with you and who will not hesitate to refer you to a specialist when one might be needed.

Education is by far the most basic tool of diabetes care. It involves learning how to take care of yourself and your diabetes, and it brings you into the decision-making process for your own health. So after you find a doctor, you'll need to add a certified diabetes educator (CDE) to your team. A certified diabetes educator is a health professional—often a nurse, registered dietitian, exercise physiologist, or pharmacist—who has additional training in helping people with diabetes to manage their disease on a day-to-day basis. Your CDE will provide you with detailed information and one-on-one guidance.

As with your doctor, the educator you choose should be someone you feel comfortable talking to and feel you can contact with questions about the practical aspects of diabetes care.

To be certified by the National Certification Board for Diabetes Educators, a health professional must have at least two years and 1,000 hours of experience in diabetes education, be currently employed in a defined role as a diabetes educator for a minimum of four hours each week, and have successfully completed a comprehensive examination covering diabetes. Your physician or health insurance plan may be able to refer you to a certified diabetes educator, or you can contact the American Association of Diabetes Educators at 1-800-338-3633 or visit their website at www.diabeteseducator.org for the names of certified diabetes educators in your area.

In addition, you should stock your diabetes care team with:

- An ophthalmologist (eye doctor), a dentist, and a podiatrist (foot doctor) experienced in treating the specific problems associated with diabetes in their respective fields
- A registered dietitian who has experience in helping people with diabetes to create and adopt a personalized meal plan and make food choices that will improve blood sugar control
- An exercise physiologist who has set up suitable exercise programs for other people with diabetes and worked with them to ensure they are executing the movements and activities safely and effectively
- A therapist, social worker, or other mental health counselor who understands the needs, concerns, and challenges of people living with a chronic disease such as diabetes

Your personal physician may be able to refer you to suitable candidates for these open spots on your diabetes care team. A family member or friend with diabetes may also have suggestions. Otherwise, you can also check the websites of various health and professional organizations; several have search functions that can provide you with the names of qualified members in your area (see the box Wanted: Experts on page 51). If you already have an established relationship with an eye doctor, dentist, or podiatrist, be sure to discuss your diabetes diagnosis with them and perhaps even put them in touch with the other members of your team so that they can collaborate on your care.

As you go about assembling your team, remember that these people work for you. You are hiring them to help you learn about diabetes, understand how it specifically affects you, and provide you with the tools to help you successfully manage your disease.

# Keep Your Team Informed

Once you've assembled your diabetes care team, it's important that you keep them on the same page by providing them with up-to-date information on your blood sugar levels, treatment plan, other medical problems, medications, and so forth. A great way to do this is by creating your own medical chart, much the way a doctor or hospital keeps a chart for each patient. This way, you can have all the information about your diabetes and your health in one place, and you can take it with you each time you meet with a member of your diabetes care team.

You'll find a list of the types of information your chart should contain in the box For the Record shown here. It is particularly crucial that your chart include a complete, accurate, and up-to-date list of all of your medications and the strength and dosage of each. Be sure to include all prescription drugs and any nonprescription medications, vitamins, minerals, supplements, and natural products you take—whether for diabetes or for any other condition/reason. It is important that each member of your care team (and any other medical professional you visit, for that matter) knows what the others have prescribed and what over-the-counter products you take so that together you can avoid dangerous interactions and overdoses.

It is also important for *you* to know what you are taking, why you are taking it, and what side effects or warning signs may occur. It is, after all, your body, and you shouldn't put anything in it that you don't understand. Be sure to note in your chart any side effects or

unusual symptoms you experience that you suspect may be connected to your medications; then be sure to inquire about them the next time you talk to the prescribing doctor.

## For Your Record

Here are the elements to include in the personal medical chart that you maintain:

A list of your medicines; their strengths; how, when, and why you take them; and who prescribed them

A list of your medical conditions and dates of diagnosis, any drug or other allergies, and all major medical events and surgeries

The names, specialties, and contact information—including emergency numbers—for all of the health care professionals you work with

Any laboratory test results as well as all handouts, booklets, or instructions given to you by members of your diabetes care team

A running list of questions you have for members of your diabetes care team (with space to record the answers)

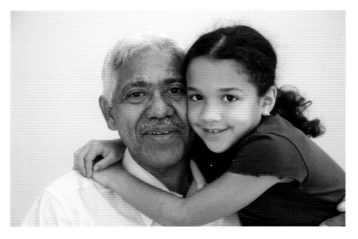

every family member—and often, close friends—to some extent. It may alter food selection and preparation and timing of shared meals. It may affect leisure time (less TV, more physical activity). It may affect finances. And it's likely to spark an array of emotions—from concern to resentment.

It's also very helpful to keep a running list of questions you have about diabetes and/or your treatment plan so that you can query the appropriate team member at your next appointment. Jot down questions or concerns in your chart as they occur to you rather than assuming you'll remember them when you meet with a team member. Often, due to the pressure of limited time or nervousness, you may forget questions that seemed so clear in your mind before you arrived for your appointment.

In addition, take time to prepare for each visit the day prior to your appointment. Be sure to bring your chart as well as your blood glucose meter and any additional logs or records you keep.

## Include Family & Friends

Diabetes is sometimes referred to as a family disease, because it tends to affect

It's also likely to prompt many questions, some you may not care to answer. ("Should you be eating that?" "Why do you have to check your blood sugar so much?" "Did you get diabetes from eating too much sugar?" "Can I catch it from you?") Still, do your best to answer them, and when you can't, ask members of your diabetes care team if they can provide you with the needed information. The more your family and friends know about your disease, the more likely they will be to accept and support your management efforts. The less they know, the more likely they will misunderstand or even unwittingly sabotage your efforts. So show off your knowledge! Teach them as much as you can about diabetes, encourage them to voice their questions and emotions, and involve them in your quest for good control. Share your treatment plan with them, explain why meal planning and blood testing are so vital to your care, tutor them on how to recognize and react to signs of hypoglycemia (which you'll learn about in Chapter 10: Beware Highs and Lows), and provide concrete suggestions for how they can support you. You might even consider encouraging them to join you in some of the healthier lifestyle choices you are making; after all, many of the diet and exercise adjustments you'll be making—like becoming more active, cutting down on junk food and other empty calories—can be beneficial for everyone, not just those who have diabetes.

At the same time, keep in mind that this is *your* diabetes, *your* health, *your* life—not theirs. If they aren't interested in joining or even supporting you, let them do what they want; it's not your job (nor is it possible, for that matter) to change the way others live their lives. All you can do is make the right choices for yourself. And if you are concerned about how others will view you for adopting a healthier lifestyle, stop worrying. Deep down,

## Wanted: Experts

American Academy of Ophthalmology
www.aao.org

American Association of Clinical Endocrinologists (AACE)
www.aace.com

American Dental Association (ADA)
www.ada.org

Academy of Nutrition and Dietetics
www.eatright.org

American Podiatric Medical Association (APMA)
www.apma.org

American Society of Exercise Physiologists (ASEP)
www.asep.org

everyone respects and admires those who make the tough choices and take good care of themselves, as long as they don't try to push their beliefs on others.

So the next time your family comes together for a birthday or holiday, don't hesitate to get up from the sofa and politely ask, "Would anyone care to join me for a walk?"

If nobody joins you, that's okay. Maybe next time someone will be inspired by what you're doing and tag along. And when you get together with your friends for a game of bridge or rummy, remember that there is no rule stating that you must consume a handful of snacks for every hand of cards. Have fun, and enjoy the camaraderie and challenge of the game. Just do so without stuffing yourself!

# Track Your Blood Sugar

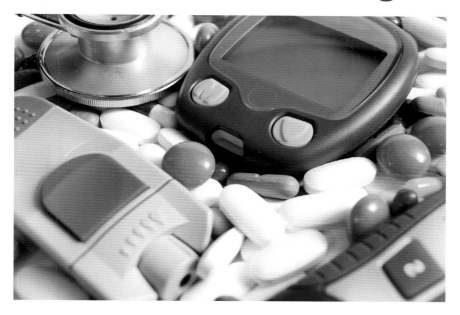

To successfully manage your diabetes and minimize your risk of suffering diabetes complications, you need to do a topnotch job of controlling your blood sugar. But how do you even know what your blood sugar level is at any particular point in time? Or how much it varies from day to day and week to week? Or whether the steps you take to get your blood sugar under control are actually working? You use two monitoring methods: individual blood sugar readings and blood tests of a substance called HbA1c.

In this chapter, we explore these two important methods for tracking your blood sugar. We look at what they can tell you about your disease management and how you can use them to improve your blood sugar control, which in turn can minimize your risk of diabetes complications. We help you set blood sugar goals that reflect a level of control appropriate for you. And we go through the practical aspects of testing your blood sugar, from selecting testing supplies and setting up a testing schedule to making sense of the results.

# Evaluating Your Control

Monitoring your blood sugar when you have diabetes or even prediabetes is very much like paying attention when you drive. You look ahead, behind, and to the sides so you can assess the conditions of the road and avoid other cars. You steal quick glances at the speedometer so you can maintain a safe speed and avoid costly tickets (and accidents). And you heed the various warning lights on the dashboard so you'll know when it's time to take your vehicle in for fuel, maintenance, or repairs.

Ignoring your blood sugar levels, on the other hand, is like driving with a blindfold on. Sooner or later, you're going to crash.

To properly manage your diabetes, you'll have to make many important choices every day. To avoid "driving blind" as you make those choices, you need to be able to "see" where your blood sugar level is and how it's been behaving in response to your "course adjustments." To gain these essential insights, you need to test your blood sugar levels often and have HbA1c tests performed regularly. Of course, you also need to have an idea of where you want to end up—in other words, where your blood sugar levels should be to give

yourself the best chance of avoiding devastating diabetes complications. And that means setting goals.

# Individual Blood Sugar Readings

Individual blood sugar readings are essential for evaluating your blood sugar control (or lack thereof). These are the readings you get by pricking your finger (or, depending on the equipment you use, an alternate site such as your arm or leg) and placing the resulting drop of blood on a test strip, which you then insert into a portable blood glucose meter. (We discuss choosing and using testing supplies later in this chapter.) The meter then measures and reports your current blood sugar level.

Regularly gathering, recording, and reviewing your individual blood sugar "numbers" in this way serves several important purposes.

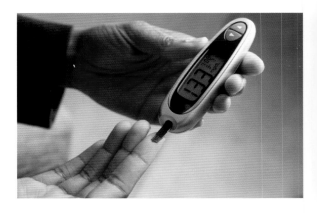

1. It provides a measuring stick for assessing your current state of blood sugar control.
2. It lets you track your progress from one point in time to another.
3. It reveals where improvements need to be made.
4. It teaches you the impact of your daily activities and choices. You can see, almost immediately, what works and what doesn't when it comes to keeping your blood sugar in a healthy range. Such prompt feedback not only provides you with a tool for tracking your control, it allows you to take action at once to bring a high or low level back into a healthier range.

Your blood sugar levels naturally vary throughout the day and from day to day, depending on a variety of factors, such as when you ate your last meal, exercised, and took any prescribed diabetes medication. By taking multiple readings each day and then averaging together all of the readings from the last one or two weeks, you can get additional insight into your level of control. Indeed, some glucose meters automatically calculate the average of your recent readings for you.

However, *quality* blood sugar control doesn't just mean having the lowest average. It also requires stability, because blood sugar readings that bounce from high to low aren't healthy, even when they result in an average that doesn't look so bad. Consider, for example, the following two people, Tim and John.

Both men have the same average blood sugar level. But look at the *variation* in John's readings in the table below: His blood sugar is high half the time and low half the time. Tim's blood sugar levels, on the other hand, are more stable and consistent, with no wild upward or downward spikes.

Too much variability in blood sugar levels can affect a person's quality of life. Having an episode of low blood sugar can be dangerous as well as uncomfortable, because it can cause symptoms such as dizziness, weakness, and rapid heartbeat; left untreated, it can quickly

| | Blood Sugar Readings | Average |
|---|---|---|
| Tim | 113, 97, 120, 135, 144, 100, 177, 83, 111 | 120 |
| John | 53, 204, 188, 67, 170, 68, 80, 202, 48 | 120 |

## Ideal Blood Sugar Ranges

| | Fasting (Wake-Up) Range | Pre-Meal Range | Post-Meal Range (1–2 Hours After Eating) |
|---|---|---|---|
| No risk of hypoglycemia* | 70–100 mg/dl | 70–120 mg/dl | <140 mg/dl |
| Low risk of hypoglycemia** | 70–120 mg/dl | 70–140 mg/dl | <160 mg/dl |
| High risk of hypoglycemia*** | 80–140 mg/dl | 80–160 mg/dl | <180 mg/dl |

*Includes those who are not taking insulin or medications that can cause hypoglycemia (glyburide, glipizide, meglitinides).*

**Includes those taking insulin once daily or oral medications that can cause hypoglycemia (glyburide, glipizide, meglitinides).*

***Includes those taking multiple insulin injections daily and those unable to detect hypoglycemia.*

lead to blurred vision, confusion, loss of consciousness, and coma (see Chapter 10: Beware Highs and Lows). Experiencing such risky lows on a regular basis is like living life on a tightrope. A high level of blood sugar, conversely, saps energy and mental focus, and frequent highs can become a real drag on the body and mind. There is also evidence that excessive variability in blood sugar levels can cause damage to blood vessels, even if the overall average is within the preferred range.

The preferred, or ideal, range for your blood sugar level depends on your current diabetes treatment regimen and how likely it is to cause hypoglycemia, or low blood sugar (see Risky Business on page 72). That ideal range also varies based on when you take a reading—your ideal range will be different after a night of fasting than it will be an hour or two after a meal, for example. You can use the table above to determine your ideal fasting, pre-meal, and post-meal ranges. Once you know them, you can assess the quality of your blood sugar control by considering how often your readings fall within the appropriate ranges.

It is not necessary for your blood sugar to be in your ideal range every time you check it. Every person who has been diagnosed with diabetes has moments of weakness when it comes to managing the disease. As a general rule, if at least 75 percent (three out of four) of your readings are in the proper range, you're doing a pretty good job of controlling your blood sugar. If more than 10 percent (one out of ten) of your readings are below your ideal range or if more than 25 percent (one out of four) are above it, you may need some additional self-management education or an adjustment to your medication regime.

Consider Irene, for example. She does not take any medication that can cause hypoglycemia, so her ideal pre-meal range is 70 to 120. The following are her pre-meal blood sugar readings for five days:

| M | Tu | W | Th | F |
|---|-----|-----|-----|-----|
| 104 | 174 | 138 | 97 | 86 |
| 225 | 126 | 125 | 101 | 99 |
| 166 | 213 | 159 | 110 | 90 |
| 113 | 98 | 79 | 185 | 143 |

Out of 20 readings, none is below her ideal range, which is good; however, 10

are above the upper limit of 120. That means 50 percent of her readings are above her ideal range. So Irene needs to work on tightening her pre-meal blood sugar control.

If your current blood sugar readings are well above your ideal ranges, it's reasonable to set temporary targets that fall between the two. For example, if you are not at risk for hypoglycemia but have blood sugars that are consistently above 200, an initial goal might be to get your readings into the 100 to 180 range. Once you've brought your sugar levels down into that target range, you can then aim for your ideal range(s).

# HbA1c Measurements

The second essential tool for gauging your blood sugar control is a test that measures glycohemoglobin A1c, often referred to as HbA1c or simply A1c. The result of this simple blood test, arranged through your doctor's office, reflects your average blood sugar level over the previous two to three months, giving you insight into your blood sugar control over a longer term.

Let's take a closer look into how this test works. Inside your red blood cells is a protein, hemoglobin, that carries oxygen from your lungs to your body's tissues.

Sugar in the blood has a tendency to glycate, or stick to, this protein, forming glycohemoglobin. Once the glucose attaches to the hemoglobin, it stays there as long as the red blood cell lives, typically two to three months. Your red blood cells don't all die at once; old ones are constantly dying, and new ones are constantly being created. So at any one time, your red blood cells are a mix of the very old, the middle aged, and the quite young.

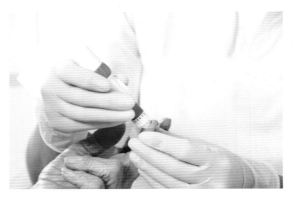

In someone without diabetes, roughly 4 to 6 percent of their hemoglobin is coated with sugar. In the person with diabetes, whose blood sugar levels are higher, more sugar attaches to the hemoglobin molecules; usually anywhere from 6 to more than 20 percent of the hemoglobin is sugar-coated. The A1c test measures this percentage. (A1c, by the way, refers to a type of glucose-coated hemoglobin that is especially suited for gauging long-term blood sugar levels.) And because some of the hemoglobin molecules in the blood are older and some newer, the A1c result provides a good estimate of how high the blood sugar has been over the past two to three months.

That's why you should ask your doctor to order an A1c test for you every three months until your sugar levels and A1c are stable and within your target ranges. Once you've reached those goals, it's usually sufficient to have the A1c test every six months, unless your doctor orders more frequent testing.

It's true that several companies sell at-home A1c test kits, but you're probably better off having a professional draw your blood and send it to a laboratory for testing. (Many doctors' offices and virtually all hospitals can do this for you.) Although the at-home kits are reasonably accurate, they require multiple steps. If any of the steps are not performed exactly right, the test will be useless and you'll have wasted your money on the cost of the kit. You may just want to let the professionals handle this test.

When you use the results from the A1c and the individual blood sugar tests you perform yourself, you get a fuller and more accurate picture of your level of control. Using the individual results alone would be like trying to judge a baseball batter's ability by looking at a day or two of single at-bats. Just as a great hitter will make an out or have a bad day sometimes, a person with good control will have the occasional high or low. So to truly gauge the player's batting skill, you need to also see his season average. And to evaluate your level of sugar control, you need to know your A1c.

To translate your A1c result into an average blood sugar level, you can use the following formula:
(A1c × 28.7) − 46.7 = average blood sugar

Or, if math isn't your thing, just use this table:

| A1c | Average Blood Sugar |
| --- | --- |
| 5% | 97 |
| 6% | 26 |
| 7% | 154 |
| 8% | 183 |
| 9% | 212 |
| 10% | 240 |
| 11% | 269 |
| 12% | 298 |
| 13% | 326 |
| 14% | 355 |

There's another reason testing A1c is so important. Research has shown it is closely linked to the risk of developing diabetic complications. The higher the A1c, the greater the risk of developing eye, kidney, nerve, and heart problems. So try to keep your A1c as near to normal as possible. In most cases, that equates to an A1c of 6 to 7 percent.

A looser A1c of 7 to 8 percent, however, may be a more appropriate target for anyone in whom an episode of hypoglycemia would be especially dangerous, including:

- Anyone who is susceptible to low blood sugar but suffers from hypoglycemia unawareness, a condition in which the individual is unable to detect the warning symptoms of a dropping blood sugar level until it is too late for them to help themselves; it can develop in people who have had diabetes for many years.
- Anyone who has significant heart disease, because the rapid heartbeat and overall physical stress placed on the body during an episode of hypoglycemia can be particularly dangerous for a person who has an already weakened heart.
- Anyone who works in an extremely high-risk profession, where experiencing dizziness, blurred vision, confusion, or loss of consciousness due to hypoglycemia could be devastating (picture a taxi driver or trucker, or a construction worker walking across a roofing beam).

- A very young child who cannot communicate symptoms of hypoglycemia.

On the other hand, a tighter A1c target of 5 to 6 percent may be appropriate for women who are pregnant or preparing to become pregnant, individuals planning for surgery, and anyone looking to slow or reverse existing diabetes complications.

Keep in mind that achieving these A1c targets may take time, especially if your current A1c is very high. Since the test is usually done every three months, it is reasonable to aim for an A1c that's one or two percentage points lower at each test.

## Your Specific Target Ranges

When you put it all together, your ideal aim is to have the lowest possible individual blood sugar and A1c levels without experiencing frequent or severe hypoglycemia. Occasional, mild episodes of low blood sugar are acceptable and not dangerous for most people with diabetes. However, if low blood sugars become too frequent (occurring more than two or three times a week) or severe (causing seizures or loss of consciousness), you'll need to ease up on your targets. So before proceeding, you need to set your own specific targets, using the information just discussed. Be sure to discuss those targets with your doctor

and other members of your diabetes care team. Set targets for the following:

- Blood sugar, fasting range (upon waking)
- Blood sugar, pre-meal range (right before eating)
- Blood sugar: post-meal range (1-2 hours after eating)
- Your Ac1 target

## Testing Your Own Blood Sugar

Okay, you've set your sights on controlling your blood sugar levels. You've even specified exactly where you want your levels to be. Now it's time to prepare for individual blood sugar testing.

## Choosing & Using Testing Supplies

To perform the individual blood sugar monitoring that is so essential to good control, you need three main supplies: a blood glucose meter, the testing strips for that meter, and a lancet or lancing device to draw the small amount of blood you'll need for testing. You will also need instruction in using the supplies you choose. Your doctor, certified diabetes educator, and/or pharmacist can give you a hands-on demonstration to ensure that you are using your equipment properly. Meter manufacturers also typically have hotlines that consumers can access in

# Common Testing Problems

| Issue | Specifics | Solution |
|---|---|---|
| Insufficient blood | If not enough blood is applied to the test area on the strip, the reading may be artificially low. | Dose the strip adequately, as the meter manufacturer instructs. If you suspect a strip contained too little blood, ignore the result and start over with a new strip. |
| Improper coding | For most meters, you must enter a code number or chip/strip for each new vial or box of strips. If the meter is not coded for that specific package of strips, the readings may be inaccurate. | Every time you begin a new box or vial of strips, code your meter according to the manufacturer's instructions. |
| Outdated strips | Using test strips that are outdated may produce inaccurate readings. | Check the expiration date before buying and again before starting a vial or box of strips. |
| Heat or humidity | Heat and humidity will cause test strips to spoil and produce false readings. | Keep your strips sealed in their packaging and away from extreme temperatures. Do not leave test strips in your vehicle! |
| Dirt/impurities | Having substances like food or grease on your finger or other test site will impact the readings. | Ensure that your test site is clean when you check your blood sugar. |

order to get answers and advice about their specific meters. Take advantage of these resources so that you can confidently and correctly measure your blood sugar levels as often as necessary for good control.

When it comes to choosing a meter, remember that quality diabetes management requires accurate and frequent blood sugar testing. Selecting a meter with the desirable qualities listed below should help make *frequent* testing less of a hassle.

- Fast (some meters take just seconds to produce a reading)
- Simple to use (fewer steps mean a quicker process and less chance for user error)
- Provides downloadable results (making it quick and easy to share your results with your diabetes care team)
- Requires very little blood (1 microliter or less is ideal)
- Easy to read (especially if you are visually impaired, choose a meter with a very large display or one that "talks")

The accuracy of just about every blood sugar meter on the market is pretty good. The values these meters produce typically fall within 15 percent of the reading a laboratory would produce on a blood sample taken at the same time. That's true, however, only if you use the correct testing technique. In the table on page 61 are some of the more common monitoring miscues, along with explanations and solutions. With the advent of alternate-site testing—using meters that can test blood taken from

## In Sight, in Mind

To encourage yourself to test your blood sugar frequently, consider keeping a meter handy wherever you tend to do the most testing. For example, you might stash meters on your bedside table, in your kitchen, at your desk or in your locker at work, in your purse or briefcase, and in your gym bag. Just avoid keeping one in your vehicle (or in a bag or tote that you leave in your vehicle for hours on end), because test strips can spoil easily at very high or low temperatures.

places other than the sensitive fingertips, such as the forearm—blood sugar testing that's virtually pain free has become a reality. However, be aware that alternate-site testing can be difficult with meters that require 1 microliter of blood or more. Also, a reading taken from the arm or leg may lag several minutes behind a reading taken from the fingertip. So if you suspect that your blood sugar is dropping quickly (after exercise or if you feel hypoglycemic) or rising quickly (after meals), blood taken from your fingertip will provide a more accurate reading than will a sample taken from an alternate site.

To make it more likely that you will perform the frequent blood sugar testing that is so conducive to good control, you may find it helpful to have more than one meter. Having multiple identical meters makes testing more convenient (you can keep one in the kitchen and one in the bedroom, for example, or one at work and one at home) and ensures that if one of your meters isn't functioning or gets misplaced, you will have an equivalent backup available. Some meter companies will even send you an extra meter at no charge in an effort to win your loyalty and keep you purchasing their test strips (they make their money off the strips). When choosing a device for drawing your blood, you'll also want to opt for features and methods that will encourage—or at least won't discourage—frequent testing. For example:

- Use the thinnest-gauge lancet you can find. (The higher the gauge, the thinner the lancet.) Thin lancets are less painful and cause less scarring than thicker lancets. Change the lancet at least once a day so the tip doesn't become dull.

- Use a lancing pen that allows you to adjust the depth of the stick, and turn it to the lightest possible setting that still produces a sufficient blood sample for your meter.
- For finger-stick testing, prick the side of your fingertip rather than the fleshy pad on the front. To obtain a sufficient blood drop after pricking, "milk" your finger by squeezing it, starting at the base and moving toward the tip.
- Opt for alternate-site testing (using your arm or leg, for example) whenever appropriate. It is almost always less painful than sticking your finger, and the readings taken at alternate sites are accurate as long as your blood sugar is not rising or dropping quickly at the time of the blood draw.

Before you go out and buy a meter at a local pharmacy, ask your doctor or diabetes educator if any free samples are available. Most meter manufacturers provide free sample meters for distribution to patients, in the hope that more patients will choose their meters and purchase their test strips for years to come. Most health insurance programs, including Medicare, Medicaid, and private insurance, cover the costs of meters, test strips, and lancets. You might want to consider using a reputable mail-order

# Why Bother Checking A1c?

Since the A1c result reflects your average blood sugar level over the previous two to three months, why not just average the results of your individual blood sugar (finger-stick) tests for that period instead? Because it doesn't work. Averaging your finger-stick readings over a three-month period almost always underestimates the true average blood sugar level as determined through the A1c test. There are several reasons why this occurs. Most people test their blood sugar before they eat, when blood sugars are at their low point, rather than after they eat, when blood sugars naturally run higher. There is also a tendency to perform the finger-stick test more frequently when blood sugars are running low, and these additional low readings tend to artificially skew the average lower. Finally, in many people, blood sugars rise in the middle of the night, a time when blood sugars are rarely checked; these highs don't get factored into an average that is calculated using only the results of individual daytime blood tests.

pharmacy or diabetes supply service; such operations will typically coordinate the insurance paperwork and ship your supplies directly to you as needed.

## Deciding How Often to Test

When it comes to blood sugar monitoring, nobody wants to do more work than is necessary. At the same time, it is essential that you gather enough data so you can assess the quality of your blood sugar control and do some fine-tuning of your management efforts. It is simply not sufficient to check your blood sugar only once a week or only when you wake up in the morning. If you check infrequently or only check at a certain time of the day, you will miss a lot of important information.

What follows are some testing recommendations that vary based on whether you have been diagnosed with type 2 diabetes or prediabetes as well as on which, if any, diabetes medication you currently use. Find the schedule that applies to your current situation, and review the schedule with your diabetes care team before proceeding. (Be sure to read the section on record keeping later in this chapter, as well.)

**For those with prediabetes or those at high risk who take no diabetes medications**

This testing schedule is for those diagnosed with prediabetes or with a high risk of developing diabetes who do not use any oral or injectable medications or insulin for their condition.

Each week, you should test your blood sugar four times: just before breakfast one day, just before lunch another day, just before dinner on a third day, and at bedtime on a fourth day. The following is an example of how you might set up this schedule:

**Sunday:** No testing required.
**Monday:** Test before breakfast.
**Tuesday:** No testing required.
**Wednesday:** Test before lunch.
**Thursday:** No testing required.
**Friday:** Test before dinner.
**Saturday:** Test at bedtime.

This schedule of testing will help you and your diabetes care team determine if your blood sugar remains in a healthy range throughout the day.

### For those with type 2 diabetes who don't take insulin
This testing schedule is for those who have been diagnosed with type 2 diabetes but who do not take any insulin for their condition. This schedule applies whether or not any oral medication or any injectable incretin (exenatide, liraglutide, or pramlintide) is also being used.

Test your blood sugar every other day as follows: just before breakfast and then one to two hours after breakfast on day one, just before lunch and then one to

two hours after lunch on day three, just before dinner and then one to two hours after dinner on day five, just before breakfast and one to two hours after breakfast on day seven, and so on. The following is an example of how you might set up this schedule:

**Monday:** Test before and one to two hours after breakfast.
**Tuesday:** No testing required.
**Wednesday:** Test before and one to two hours after lunch.
**Thursday:** No testing required.
**Friday:** Test before and one to two hours after dinner.
**Saturday:** No testing required.
**Sunday:** Test before and one to two hours after breakfast.
**Monday:** No testing required.

This testing schedule will allow you and your diabetes care team to see if your blood sugar remains normal before and after each of your meals. The wake-up and other pre-meal readings indicate whether your body is able to make enough of its own basal insulin, the baseline amount of insulin needed to offset the sugar that's naturally released by the liver between meals to maintain basic bodily functions. The after-meal readings indicate whether your pancreas can make enough bolus insulin, the additional burst of insulin needed at mealtimes to offset the carbohydrates from a meal.

**For those with type 2 diabetes who take long-acting but not rapid-acting insulin**
This testing schedule is for those who have been diagnosed with type 2 diabetes who are currently taking long-acting insulin (glargine, detemir, or NPH) but no rapid-acting (lispro, aspart, or glulisine) or pre-mixed (50/50, 70/30, or 75/25) insulin. This schedule applies whether or not any oral medication or injectable incretin (exenatide, liraglutide, or pramlintide) is also being used.

## More than Just Numbers

In recent years, a number of researchers have questioned the value of home blood sugar monitoring for people with type 2 diabetes. In each of the studies, however, a key element was neglected—teaching people to interpret their own information. Virtually every qualified diabetes specialist recommends home blood sugar monitoring for their patients with diabetes, because they recognize the value of home testing; they realize that intelligent adjustments to treatment can be made—by patients and/or their diabetes care team—when the test results are analyzed on a regular basis.

Test your blood sugar at least twice a day, six days a week, as follows: On the first day, test just before and one to two hours after breakfast; on the second day, test just before and one to two hours after lunch; on the third day, test just before and one to two hours after dinner and also at bedtime if it follows dinner by more than three hours; and on days four through six, repeat the schedule from days one through three. Take a break from testing on the last day of each week. The following is an example of how you might set up this schedule:

**Monday:** Test before and one to two hours after breakfast.
**Tuesday:** Test before and one to two hours after lunch.
**Wednesday:** Test before and one to two hours after dinner and at bedtime (if it's more than three hours after dinner).
**Thursday:** Test before and one to two hours after breakfast.
**Friday:** Test before and one to two hours after lunch.
**Saturday:** Test before and one to two hours after dinner and at bedtime (if it's more than three hours after dinner).
**Sunday:** No testing required.

This testing schedule will allow you and your diabetes care team to see if your blood sugar remains normal before and after each of your meals.

**For those with type 2 diabetes who take premixed insulin twice a day**

This testing schedule is for those diagnosed with type 2 diabetes who currently inject premixed insulin (50/50, 70/30, or 75/25) twice each day rather than injecting long-acting (glargine, detemir, or NPH) and/or rapid-acting (lispro, aspart, or glulisine) insulin separately. This schedule applies whether or not any oral medication or injectable incretin (exenatide, liraglutide, or pramlintide) is also being used.

Each day of the week, test your blood sugar upon waking (before breakfast), at midday (before lunch), late in the afternoon (before dinner), and at bedtime. Also, as part of your weekly testing regimen, test your blood sugar one to two hours after breakfast on one day, one to two hours after lunch on another day, and one to two hours after dinner on a third day. The following is a sample schedule:

**Sunday:** Test before breakfast, before lunch, before dinner, and at bedtime.
**Monday:** Test before breakfast, one to two hours after breakfast, before lunch, before dinner, and at bedtime.
**Tuesday:** Test before breakfast, before lunch, before dinner, and at bedtime.
**Wednesday:** Test before breakfast, before lunch, one to two hours after lunch,

## If You Have Type 1

Blood sugar testing is absolutely essential if you have been diagnosed with type 1 diabetes. For you, it's truly a matter of life and death. Your testing schedule may be similar to the one described in the text for people with type 2 diabetes who take insulin at each meal, but you must work with your diabetes care team to determine the timing and frequency of daily testing that is most appropriate for you, based on a variety of factors, including your current level of control.

before dinner, and at bedtime.
**Thursday:** Test before breakfast, before lunch, before dinner, and at bedtime.
**Friday:** Test before breakfast, before lunch, before dinner, one to two hours after dinner, and at bedtime.
**Saturday:** Test before breakfast, before lunch, before dinner, and at bedtime.

The pre-meal checks allow evaluation of the effectiveness of your insulin doses, while the post-meal checks help determine the optimal timing of your two daily injections.

**For those with type 2 diabetes who take insulin at each meal**

This testing schedule is for those diagnosed with type 2 diabetes who currently inject rapid-acting insulin (lispro, aspart, or glulisine) at each meal and use long-acting insulin (glargine, detemir, or NPH) to cover their basal insulin needs. (No premixed insulin is used.) This schedule applies whether or not any oral medication or injectable incretin (exenatide, liraglutide, or pramlintide) is also being used.

Each day of the week, test your blood sugar just before every meal; just before your afternoon snack; just before your evening snack or, if you don't eat an evening snack, just before going to bed; prior to exercise; and before driving. Also, one day a week, test your blood sugar one to two hours after breakfast; on another day of the week, test one to two hours after lunch; and on a third day, test one to two hours after dinner. The following is a sample schedule:

**Sunday:** Test upon waking; before lunch; before your afternoon snack; before dinner; before your evening snack or at bedtime; and before exercising or driving.
**Monday:** Test upon waking; one to two hours after breakfast; before lunch; before your afternoon snack; before dinner; before your evening snack or at bedtime; and before exercising or driving.
**Tuesday:** Test upon waking, before lunch,

before your afternoon snack, before dinner, before your evening snack or at bedtime, and before exercising or driving.
**Wednesday:** Test upon waking; before lunch; one to two hours after lunch; before your afternoon snack; before dinner; before your evening snack or at bedtime; and before exercising or driving.
**Thursday:** Test upon waking; before lunch; before your afternoon snack; before dinner; before your evening snack or at bedtime; and before exercising or driving.
**Friday:** Test upon waking; before lunch; before your afternoon snack; before dinner; one to two hours after dinner;

## Help at Your Fingertips

If you ever have trouble with your blood sugar meter, call the toll-free number located on the back of the machine. Every meter manufacturer offers a 24-hour toll-free hotline for its meter customers. Call the hotline if you have questions about proper testing procedure, are concerned about the accuracy of any readings, experience difficulties with the meter, discover that a part is missing or broken, or want to learn how to use any of your meter's advanced features (including memory recall or downloading).

before your evening snack or at bedtime; and before exercising or driving.

**Saturday:** Test upon waking; before lunch; before your afternoon snack; before dinner; before your evening snack or at bedtime; and before exercising or driving.

The pre-meal tests are necessary because they allow you and your diabetes care team to evaluate the effectiveness of your insulin doses. The pre-driving and pre-exercise tests are for safety purposes. The post-meal tests help you and your team determine the optimal timing of your insulin doses.

# Recording & Analyzing Your Results

To make your testing worthwhile, you need to review and learn from your results. By keeping organized and accurate records of your blood sugar tests and analyzing them on a regular basis, you can gain tremendous insight into your diabetes management program.

At its most basic, your record keeping system should include the date and time of every blood sugar test and the results you obtained from each one. As long as your blood sugar readings are consistently within your target ranges, it is not usually necessary to keep track of anything else. But if some of the readings are above

or below target, it becomes necessary to figure out why.

Was a high or low reading caused by the consumption of too much or too little food? The wrong type, dose, or timing of medication? Was it due to an unusual amount of physical activity? Maybe stress or illness? Every time you use your records to make a sensible adjustment to your treatment regimen (whether in the type, amount, or timing of food, physical activity, or medication), your blood sugar control will get a little bit better.

If you need to figure out why your blood sugar levels are straying outside their target ranges, you will need to record other information in addition to your test results. The same is true if your treatment regimen calls for injecting insulin at mealtimes, an approach that requires you to account for meals and physical activity in determining the correct dose of insulin. In either situation, you will need to record the major factors that influence blood sugar levels, including:

- The type, dose, and timing of any diabetes medication (whether it's oral medication, noninsulin injection, and/or insulin)
- The grams of carbohydrate consumed in each meal and snack (Carb counting will be explained in detail in the next chapter.)

| | Before Breakfast | After Breakfast | Before Lunch | After Lunch | Before Dinner | After Dinner |
|---|---|---|---|---|---|---|
| Mon 3/3 | 95 | 166 | | | | |
| Wed 3/5 | | | 87 | 144 | | |
| Fri 3/7 | | | | | 77 | 158 |
| Sun 3/9 | 99 | 190 | | | | |
| Tue 3/9 | | | 80 | 133 | | |
| Thu 3/13 | | | | | 100 | 202 |
| Sat 3/15 | 81 | 175 | | | | |

- The type and length of exercise and other physical activities performed, such as housework, yard work, shopping, and extended walking
- Stresses that tend to affect blood sugar levels, such as physical illness, menstrual cycles, emotional events, and hypoglycemic episodes.

Your log sheets need not be fancy. A ruled notebook with columns and headers penciled in by hand will work just fine.

Learning how to interpret your self-monitoring records is also essential. Otherwise, your records are nothing more than pieces of paper covered with numbers. To get the most from your record keeping, it helps to organize the information so it will be easy to analyze. One way is to line up several days' data in columns so that you can detect blood sugar patterns that occur at particular times of day. If you notice that your blood sugar levels are consistently high or low at a certain point each day, it is easy to make the right kind of adjustment to bring it back in line.

To see how this works, consider the table on this page, which shows two weeks of blood sugar test results for Wendy. Wendy has type 2 diabetes and is currently taking no insulin or other

| | Before Breakfast | After Breakfast | Before Lunch | After Lunch | Before Dinner | After Dinner | Bedtime |
|---|---|---|---|---|---|---|---|
| Mon 3/3 | 188 | 131 | | | | | |
| Tue 3/4 | | | 102 | 122 | | | |
| Wed 3/5 | | | | | 87 | 128 | 104 |
| Thu 3/6 | 211 | 135 | | | | | |
| Fri 3/7 | | | 110 | 114 | | | |
| Sat 3/8 | | | | | 85 | 99 | 98 |

medication for her diabetes. Her target blood sugar ranges are:

Fasting (before breakfast): 70-100
Before other meals: 70-120
After meals: <140

Notice how Wendy's pre-meal blood sugars are consistently near normal, but her after-meal readings are generally above her target range. It looks as though Wendy needs to work on managing her post-meal blood sugar, possibly through reduced carb intake at meals, some physical activity after meals, or the addition of a mealtime medication.

Now consider the results shown on this page for Toni. Toni is taking long-acting insulin once a day and oral diabetes medication at each meal. Her target blood sugar ranges are:

Fasting (before breakfast): 70-120
Before other meals: 70-140
After meals: <160

Toni's pre- and post-meal blood sugars are all pretty close to her targets, except for her level first thing in the morning. Toni's dose of long-acting insulin likely needs to be increased, or she needs to reduce her late-night snacking.

When you first begin testing, recording, and analyzing your own blood sugar levels, you should review your readings every couple of weeks. If they are fairly stable and within their target ranges, then monthly record reviews should be enough. But if you detect a pattern of readings that are out of range (above or below), bring them to the attention of your diabetes care team. Working with your team, you should be able to develop an effective solution for any control problem. And as your experience grows, there will likely come a time when you will be able to determine for yourself what minor adjustments to make in your treatment regimen to bring any errant levels back where they belong. (Even then, you'll need regular check-ins with your diabetes care team.)

## Continuous Glucose Monitoring

Another tool in diabetes management technology is continuous glucose monitoring (CGM). Several systems are now available (by prescription) that provide blood sugar readings once every one to five minutes and emit warnings when the sugar level is heading for a high or low. These systems use a sensor, a thin metallic filament inserted just below the skin, to detect sugar in the fluid between fat cells. They come with a spring-loaded device that makes inserting

the sensor quick and relatively painless. The information from the sensor is transmitted via radio signals to a receiver that looks like a cell phone. The receiver displays charts, graphs, and an estimate of the current blood sugar level. The transmitter and receiver are reusable, although the sensor filament must be replaced every few days or so, depending on the specific system and the body's ability to tolerate the filament.

## Risky Business

Many older diabetes medications force the pancreas to secrete extra insulin regardless of the blood sugar level and can therefore cause hypoglycemia, or low blood sugar. These medications include the ones listed below as well as any combination pills that contain any of these medications:

- tolbutamide (Orinase)
- acetohexamide (Dymelor)
- tolazamide (Tolinase)
- chlorpropamide (Diabinese)
- glipizide (Glucotrol)
- glyburide (Diabeta, Micronase, Glynase)
- glimepiride (Amaryl)
- gliclazide (Diamicron)
- repaglinide (Prandin)
- nateglinide (Starlix)

CGM devices are generally accurate to within about 15 percent of most finger-stick readings. They generate line graphs that depict sugar levels over the past several hours, allowing the user to detect trends and predict where blood sugar is headed. They use either vibration or a beeping noise to alert the wearer to impending high and low blood sugar levels. And computer or internet-based programs allow for detailed analysis of blood sugar levels over longer intervals of time.

Comparing finger-stick blood sugar testing to CGM is like comparing a photograph to a movie. CGM shows change and movement. It illustrates how virtually everything in daily life influences blood sugar levels. Used just once or twice, CGM can offer insight into the effectiveness of an individual's current diabetes management program. Worn on an ongoing basis, CGM makes it easier to keep blood sugars in range on a consistent basis, and there is less risk of experiencing dangerous highs or lows.

Of course, CGM does have its drawbacks. It can be costly, and many health insurance plans resist covering it for people with type 2 diabetes. In addition, a CGM system requires some maintenance and technical know-how, and it's not always the most accurate testing method. It also still requires the user to enter the results from periodic finger-stick readings for calibration purposes, and improperly calibrating the device can lead to erroneous readings. However, if CGM sounds interesting to you, don't hesitate to talk to your diabetes care team to gather more information about it and see if it's right for you.

# Fight Diabetes with Food

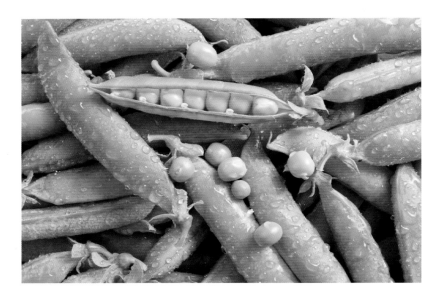

No approach to tight control of blood sugar and diabetes would be complete without a sound eating plan. A well-designed eating plan will reduce the risks of hypoglycemia and diabetes complications, control weight, and provide the nutrients you need to keep your body running in top form. A well-designed eating plan will also be something you can sustain over time.

There are three main factors you need to keep your body running in top form: **Carbohydrates.** They have the greatest immediate impact on your blood sugar level. Determining a safe and healthy amount of carbohydrates for you to consume each day is the bedrock of a comprehensive meal plan.
**Glycemic index.** In many cases the rate at which you digest is just as important as what you digest.
**Calories.** You need to balance your energy intake against your energy expenditure.

When you understanding these factors and take them into account when making your food choices, you'll be that much closer to bringing your blood sugar under control.

# Carbohydrates

Carbohydrates include simple sugars as well as complex carbs. Simple sugars include sucrose (table sugar), fructose (fruit sugar), lactose (milk sugar), and corn syrup. Foods rich in simple carbs include fruit, fruit juice, regular soda, candy, chocolate, cookies, cakes, pastries, milk, ice cream, yogurt, sports drinks, honey, syrup, and jelly.

Complex carbs are better known as starches. You can think of a simple sugar as an individual railroad car and a starch

as a bunch of cars hooked together to make a train. Most starches are composed of many sugar molecules linked together. Food rich in starches, or complex carbs, include potatoes, rice, pasta, cereal, oatmeal, bread, pizza, tortillas, bagels, beans, corn, pretzels, chips, and popcorn.

The carbs you eat are converted by your body into glucose, the sugar that circulates through your bloodstream to nourish your body's cells. That blood sugar is your body's primary fuel. To get the sugar out of your bloodstream and into your body's cells, your pancreas

## No-Carb No-No

Everyone needs some carbohydrates in their diet. Carbs are the primary source of the glucose that cells use for energy, and the body easily turns carbs into blood sugar. If you consume no carbs, your body is forced to dismantle valuable protein (the stuff muscles are made of) for fuel, something it prefers not to do. In the absence of carbs, your body also begins breaking down fat for fuel, but the byproducts (called ketones) that result can, over time, throw off your body's acid-base balance and damage your liver and kidneys. Meanwhile, you are left vulnerable to bouts of lethargy and low blood sugar.

# REASONABLE DAILY CARBOHYDRATE INTAKE FOR PEOPLE WITH (OR AT RISK OF) TYPE 2 DIABETES:

| | Short Stature | | Medium Stature | | Tall Stature | |
|---|---|---|---|---|---|---|
| | Male | Female | Male | Female | Male | Female |
| Fairly Inactive | 120–140g | 110–130g | 140–160g | 120–140g | 180–210g | 140–160g |
| Moderately Active | 160–190g | 130–160g | 190–220g | 140–170g | 220–250g | 160–190g |
| Very Active | 180–220g | 150–190g | 220–260g | 160–200g | 250–300g | 180–220g |

produces insulin. When you consume large amounts of carbohydrate, it places a heavy workload on the pancreas. And when you eat carbs that digest very quickly, the pancreas must pump out insulin at a furious rate to keep up with the sudden rush of sugar into the bloodstream. In people who are insulin resistant or who have a pancreas that has a hard time keeping up, there simply may not be enough insulin produced to keep the blood sugar level from going too high.

Consuming too much carbohydrate will also contribute to weight gain, which makes the body's cells even more insulin resistant.

For many years, doctors and others advised people with diabetes to avoid simple sugars as much as possible. However, the current understanding is that from the standpoint of blood sugar control, it doesn't matter if the carbs you eat are simple sugars or complex carbs (starches). Both will raise blood sugar by the same amount. If you eat a cup of pasta that contains 60 grams of complex carbohydrate, that will raise your blood sugar just as much as if you drink a can of regular soda containing 60 grams of simple sugars. Both will raise your blood sugar level pretty fast.

In other words, if you're looking for information about how a particular food will affect your blood sugar, focus on its total carbohydrate content more than its sugar content.

So how much carbohydrate should you eat? That depends on many factors, including your level of physical activity, your height, and the amount of weight you want to lose. It's something you should discuss with a registered dietitian (R.D.) who is also a certified

## Add to Subtract

In weight loss terms, you're said to have "hit a plateau" when you've reached a certain weight and can't seem to lose any more pounds. When this happens, sometimes the cure is to take in more rather than fewer calories. How could that be? If you take in too few calories, your metabolism (the rate at which your body burns calories to fuel its processes and activities) may actually slow down. The body thinks it is starving and lowers its metabolic rate to conserve what few calories are coming in. So if you've hit a plateau, try taking in a few more calories each day to see if your metabolic rate resets and you begin losing pounds again.

| Exchange Group—see page 80 | Carbohydrate | Protein | Fat |
|---|---|---|---|
| **Bread:** 1 slice bread; ¾ cup corn flakes; 6 saltine crackers; ½ cup noodles | Lots (15g) | Little (3g) | Little (1g) |
| **Fruit:** ½ cup orange juice; 1 small apple; ½ banana; 1 cup watermelon | Lots (15g) | None (0g) | None (0g) |
| **Vegetable:** ⅓ cup cooked carrots; ½ cup fresh peas; 1 cup spinach; ½ cup canned tomato | Little (5g) | Little (2g) | None (0g) |
| **Milk:** 1 cup milk or unsweetened yogurt | Moderate (12g) | Lots (8g) | Varies (1–8g) |
| **Meat:** 1 oz. meat, cheese, or cold cuts; 2 tbs. peanut butter | None (0g) | Lots (7g) | Varies (3–8g) |
| **Fat:** 1 tsp. butter; 1 strip bacon; 1 tsp. vegetable oil; 2 tbs. sour cream | None (0g) | None (0g) | Lots (5g) |

diabetes educator (C.D.E.) or at least has experience counseling people with diabetes. (See Chapter 3: Enlist Help for information on adding a dietitian to your diabetes care team.) Check your health insurance plan first, as many plans will cover all or part of the cost of meeting with a dietitian at least once. Even if they don't, it's still well worth the cost, because it will help you improve your blood sugar control. That, in turn, will help you prevent, postpone, or slow diabetes complications, which can prove costly to both your wallet and your health further down the road.

Until you can meet with a dietitian and develop an individualized plan, you can use some general carbohydrate recommendations to get started. First, you need to estimate how much carbohydrate you should have in a typical day. The amounts shown in the table on page 76 provide a reasonable starting range of intake—based on gender, height/body size, and activity level— for people who have or are at risk of developing type 2 diabetes.

Once you have an idea of how much total carbohydrate to consume daily, you need to know how to distribute it throughout the day. Let's say you're shooting for about 160 grams of carbohydrate a day. You don't want to consume that all at once, which would put too much strain on your body's ability to regulate blood sugar following a meal. Instead, divide your carbs among at least three meals and one or two snacks per day.

For example, if you have 160 grams of carbohydrate to "spend" for the day, you could have 30 grams for breakfast, 45 for lunch, 20 in an afternoon snack, 45 for dinner, and 20 in an evening snack. Remember that the goal is to keep your total carbohydrate intake within a reasonable range. Avoid flooding your bloodstream with too much glucose at any one sitting.

# Carbohydrate Counting Techniques

Keeping your daily carbohydrate intake in a reasonable range is important for regaining control of your blood sugar levels, but it requires you to have a system for quantifying the amount of carbohydrate in the foods you eat— in other words, a technique for *carb counting.* By counting carbs, people in the early stages of type 2 diabetes can avoid overworking the pancreas. For those in more advanced stages of diabetes, carb counting allows them to match insulin doses to the food being eaten. What follows are discussions of the primary carb counting methods.

# No Label? No Problem.

Nutrient labels make carb counting easy, but only if there's a label on every food you eat. Unpackaged foods, such as fresh fruits and vegetables, some baked goods, fast foods, and made-to-order foods, typically do not carry labels. For these, you need to refer to a printed or electronic nutrient guide that lists the serving size and the per-serving amounts of total carb, fiber, and calories for unlabeled foods. Fortunately, you can access the U.S. Government's free nutrient database at ndb.nal.usda.gov. You can use the site's search function to view the carb and calorie counts for specific serving sizes of thousands upon thousands of foods. You may also be able to find online nutrient listings for the foods served at fast-food and sit-down restaurant chains by typing the name of the chain into a search engine. Many fast-food restaurants also have printed nutrient listings available in-store for customers.

## 1. Carb Exchanging

One of the most basic methods for counting carbs involves converting food types into grams of carbohydrate. It is based on the traditional, more complex diabetic "Exchange System," in which foods are grouped by their typical nutrient content. For example, one slice of bread counts as one "starch." A small apple is counted as one "fruit."

You may have heard people with diabetes say they get "three breads at breakfast, four at lunch, four at dinner, and two at bedtime." In this context, a "bread" may mean either a slice of bread or a food similar in carbohydrate, fat, and protein content to a slice of bread. A slice of bread has lots of carbs (15 grams per serving), with a small amount of protein and fat. The same can be said of a half cup spaghetti, three cups popcorn, or 1/3 cup corn. In other words, three cups of popcorn can be "exchanged" for a slice of bread because it contains about the same carb count.

The same holds true for the other exchanges. Just like a typical piece of meat, a "meat" exchange has very few carbs, a lot of protein, and a moderate-to-high amount of fat.

| | |
|---|---|
| 1 "Bread" Exchange | = 15 grams carb |
| 1 "Fruit" Exchange | = 15 grams carb |
| 1 "Milk" Exchange | = 12 grams carb |
| 1 "Vegetable" Exchange | = 5 grams carb |
| 1 "Meat" Exchange | = 0 grams carb |
| 1 "Fat" Exchange | = 0 grams carb |

The table on page 78 shows examples of foods in each exchange group and their approximate per-serving nutrient content.

The list on page 80 shows you how many grams of carbohydrate you get from a single selection in each exchange. To figure out how much carbohydrate you're having in a meal, add up the grams of carbohydrate you are getting from each exchange. A meal of two breads (2 × 15), two fruits (2 × 15), a milk (1 × 12), and three meats (3 × 0) supplies a total of 72 grams of carbohydrate. Just be sure that your portions match the definition of a single serving in each food's exchange. For example, a small apple counts as a single "fruit" exchange, but if the apple you are eating is medium or large, it counts as 1½ or 2 "fruit" exchanges, so your carb calculation needs to reflect this. You'll find a more detailed exchange list at the back of this book.

## 2. Label Reading

When it comes to carb counting, food labels can be your best friend. The U.S. Food and Drug Administration (FDA) requires all packaged and processed foods to list pertinent nutrient information such as total grams of carbohydrate, grams of sugar, and grams of fiber in a single serving of the food. Fiber is a unique type of carbohydrate in that it passes through the body undigested and thus adds no calories and has little effect on blood sugar. Many foods contain little or no fiber, so for them, the total carbohydrate figure on the label can be used for carb counting. For foods that do contain fiber, you'll need to subtract the grams of fiber from the grams of total carbohydrate to arrive at the number of carbohydrate grams to use in carb counting.

Let's take a look at an example. The Nutrition Facts label shown here is for a food item that contains 29 grams of total carbohydrate per serving. The 16 grams of sugar are already included in the total carbohydrate figure, so there is no need

## Nutrition Facts

Serving Size ½ cup
Servings Per Container 8

Amount Per Serving

| Calories 125 | Calories from fat 18 |
|---|---|

| | % Daily Value* |
|---|---|
| Total Fat 2g | 4% |
| Saturated Fat 0g | 0% |
| Trans Fat 0g | 0% |
| Cholesterol 0mg | 0% |
| Sodium 120mg | 5% |
| Total Carbohydrate 29g | 10% |
| Dietary Fiber 3g | |
| Sugars 16g | |
| Protein 2g | |

* Percent Daily Values are based on a 2,000 calorie diet.

to count them separately. A single serving also contains 3 grams of fiber, which you do need to subtract from the 29 grams of total carbohydrate, leaving you with 26 grams of digestible carbs to include in your carb count that day.

It's also important to be sure the amount you eat matches the serving size listed on the label. If your portion is smaller or larger than the listed serving size, you need to adjust the carbohydrate total accordingly. In the example above, for instance, the serving size is 1/2 cup. If you consume a full cup, which is twice the amount of a single serving, you need to double the 26 grams of digestible carbs, for a grand total of 52 grams to include in your carb count.

## 3. Portion Conversion

This highly practical (but not as precise) technique for counting carbs makes use of portion estimation and is particularly useful when you're having a complex meal, dining out, or enjoying foods that vary in size. *Portion estimation* involves using a common object such as your fist, a tennis ball, or a milk carton to estimate the volume of a food. Once you've estimated the volume of your portion in this way, you then convert the volume measurement into a carb count based on the typical amount of carbohydrate per unit volume for that type of food.

### A Handy Measure

When using portion conversion to count carbs, the fist of an average adult is considered equal to one cup. To find out if your own fist is roughly equal to one cup, take a large measuring cup or bowl and fill it halfway with water. Then immerse your fist completely in the water, and see how much the water level rises.

Confused yet? Don't be. Here's an example that should make this very clear: If you know that one cup of fruit juice contains about 30 grams of carbohydrate, and you are having a portion of juice equal to 1½ cups, you are having 30 × 1.5, or 45, grams of carbohydrate. The key to making this method work is to obtain a fairly accurate size estimate for each food portion you consume. Below are some common "measuring devices" that can be used for physically "seeing" or mentally "visualizing" portion volumes:

Adult's palm = approx. 4" diameter
Adult's spread hand = approx. 8" diameter
Average adult's fist = approx. 1 cup
Child's fist = approx. ½ cup
Cupped hand = approx. ½ cup
Half-pint milk = 1 cup
Large handful = approx. 1 cup

Soda can (12 oz.) = 1½ cups
Tennis ball = approx. ¾ cup

Keep in mind that volume consists of three dimensions: length, width, *and* height. The thickness or "tallness" of the food item should be taken into account when estimating the volume. Also, be sure to count only the portion that you are actually going to eat. The rind or peel on fruit, for example, should not be counted, nor should potato skins or bread crusts if you don't plan to eat them.

Below are approximate carb counts for standard portion sizes:
Bread, dense (bagel/soft pretzel) = 50g cup
Bread/long sandwich roll = 8g/inch
Cake/muffin/pie = 50g/cup
Cereal, cold = 25g/cup
Chips = 15g/cup

Cookie = 20g/4" diameter
Fruit, summer = 20g/cup
Fruit, winter = 25g/cup
Ice cream = 35g/cup
Juice = 30g/cup
Milk = 12g/cup
Pancake, thin = 8g/4" diameter
Pasta, plain = 35g/cup
Pizza = 40g/8" diameter
Popcorn = 5g/cup
Potato = 30g/cup
Pretzels = 25g/cup
Rice, "sticky" = 75g/cup
Rice, instant = 50g/cup
Rolls = 25g/cup
Salad = 5g/cup
Soda, nondiet = 30g/cup
Sports drink = 15g/cup
Tortilla = 15g/8" diameter
Vegetables, cooked = 10g/cup
Vegetables, raw = 5g/cup

## Rules of Thumb

- High-fiber foods raise blood sugar more slowly than low-fiber foods do.
- High-fat foods raise blood sugar more slowly than low-fat foods do.
- Solids raise blood sugar more slowly than liquids do.
- Cold foods raise blood sugar more slowly than hot foods do.
- Unripe foods raise blood sugar more slowly than ripe foods do.
- Raw foods raise blood sugar more slowly than cooked foods do

Here's how you would make portion conversion work: According to the list above, the fist of an average-size adult is roughly equal to a one-cup portion. If a cup of instant rice contains 50 grams of carbohydrate and you eat 1½ fist-size portions of instant rice, you are consuming about 75 grams of carbohydrate. If you eat three large handfuls of chips, you are consuming about three cups worth, and since one cup of chips contains 15 grams of carbohydrate, your three cups (or large handfuls) of chips are supplying you with about 45 grams of carbs.

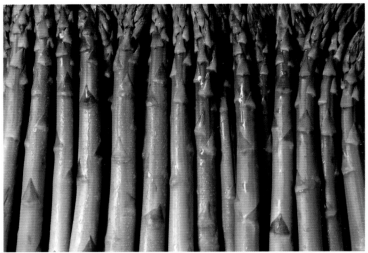

The best way to fine-tune your portion estimation skills is through practice. Estimate the volume of a food item (using your fist or another item of known volume for comparison), and then either look up the exact volume on the food's label or place it in a measuring cup. Doing this repeatedly will train your eye and your mind to estimate portions accurately.

## 4. Carb Factors

Using carb factors involves weighing a portion of food on a scale and then multiplying the weight of the food in grams by its carb factor (which represents the percentage of the food's weight that is carbohydrate). Doing so will produce a fairly precise carb count for that portion of food. For example, apples have a carb factor of .13, which means that 13 percent of an average apple's weight is carbohydrate. If an apple without its core weighs 120 grams, the carb content is 120 × .13, or 15.6, grams.

Carb factors should only take into account the food that will actually be eaten. Foods should be weighed *without* the core, peel, rind, skin, seeds, packaging, crust, or any other part that will not actually be consumed.

Carb factors are most helpful with foods eaten at home (nobody expects you to carry a scale everywhere you go), where the food may be an odd shape, the food density can vary considerably, or the

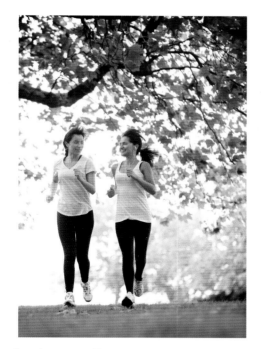

the digestible carbs you consume will eventually be converted by your body into blood glucose, some make the transition much faster than others. The rate at which different carbs are converted into blood glucose can be compared using something called the Glycemic Index (GI). A food's GI score, therefore, is another factor to take into account when considering the effect a food will have on blood sugar.

The GI ranks foods on a scale from 0 to 100. At the top, with a score of 100, is pure glucose (listed as dextrose on package labels). Other foods are ranked in comparison to the absorption rate of pure glucose. (There's a list of GI scores for many common foods at the end of the book.)

food is actually a mixture of several foods. Examples include beef stew, homemade breads/pastries, and baked potatoes.

To figure the carb factor for packaged food, check the food label for the total grams of carbohydrates and the weight of a serving. Divide the first number by the second. For example, if a serving of pastry contains 60 grams of carb and weighs 150 grams, its carb factor is 60 ÷ 150, or .40. You could then weigh any size portion of that pastry and multiply by .40 to determine the exact carb count.

## Glycemic Index

Now that you understand carb counting, it's time for a revelation: Not all carbs are created equal. While virtually all of

What the score actually represents is the percentage of a food's carbohydrate content that turns into blood glucose within the two hours after the food is eaten. Foods with a high GI score (above 70) tend to be digested and converted into glucose the fastest, producing a significant peak in blood sugar 30 to 45 minutes after they are eaten. Foods with a moderate GI score of 45 to 70 digest a bit slower, resulting in a less pronounced peak in blood sugar approximately one to two hours after they are eaten. Foods with a low GI score (below 45) have a

Below are some commonsense substitutions you can try:

| MEAL | HIGH-GI CHOICES | LOWER-GI CHOICES |
|------|-----------------|------------------|
| Breakfast | Typical cold cereal, bagel, toast, waffle, pancake, corn muffin | High-fiber cereal, oatmeal, yogurt, whole fruit, milk, bran muffin |
| Lunch | Sandwich made with white or whole-wheat bread, French fries, tortillas, canned pasta | Chili, pumpernickel bread, corn, carrots, raw salad vegetables |
| Dinner | Rice, rolls, white potato, canned vegetables | Sweet potato, pasta, beans, fresh or steamed vegetables |
| Snacks | Pretzels, chips, crackers, cake, donut | Popcorn, whole fruit, frozen yogurt |

slow, gradual effect on the blood sugar level: The peak is usually quite modest and may take several hours to occur.

White bread, for example, has a GI score of 71, and an apple has a score of 38. Their respective scores tell you that the white bread will raise blood sugar much faster than the apple will. Interestingly, wheat bread, with a score of 68, raises blood sugar almost as quickly as white bread does. On the other hand, sweet potatoes, with a score of 44, are much slower to raise blood sugar than are baked white potatoes, which have a score of 85. So it's not always easy to correctly guess a food's score.

Still, most starchy foods have a relatively high GI score: They are easily digested and quickly converted into blood sugar. Exceptions include starches found in legumes (dried beans and peas) and pasta. Foods that contain dextrose tend to rank very high on the Index. Fructose (fruit sugar) and lactose (milk sugar) are

If you've chosen the healthy path to weight loss and have begun including daily exercise along with dietary changes, the bathroom scale may not reflect all the progress you're making, because you may be losing more fat than pounds. Many forms of exercise can help you to burn off pounds of unsightly, unhealthy body fat, but some can also add lean mass, or lean weight, by building toned, calorie-burning muscle and denser, stronger bones. So rather than using the scale alone to gauge your progress, you should also measure your chest, waist, and hips with a tape measure or ask a fitness professional to measure your body fat percentage. These additional measures will provide you with "hard" evidence that you're losing fat and building muscle.

converted into blood sugar more slowly than are most starches. Table sugar (sucrose) has a moderate GI score because it contains a combination of quickly converted glucose and more slowly converted fructose. Foods that contain fiber or large amounts of fat tend to have lower GI scores than do low-fat foods and foods without fiber.

Why care about GI scores? Because the effect that different foods have on your blood sugar is what really matters. In general, consuming primarily low-GI foods tends to make blood sugar easier to control. These foods enhance the feeling of fullness and help curb appetite (both great for weight control). In a person who is insulin resistant or whose pancreas has difficulty making large amounts of insulin all at once, low-GI foods are better tolerated. When low-GI foods are eaten, the pancreas is able to control blood sugar by releasing insulin gradually; it doesn't have to produce a huge burst of insulin to keep up with a sudden flood of sugar into the bloodstream. Eating a diet of slowly digesting (low-GI) foods simply works better for people with diabetes because it eases the workload on the pancreas, prevents post-meal "spikes" in blood sugar, and provides a satisfying form of slow-burning fuel.

## Calories & Weight Loss

When you consume more calories than your body uses for fuel, the extra calories have to go somewhere. Typically, they get stored as fat. That fat can only be eliminated if you start to burn more calories than you take in. It doesn't matter where the calories come from, whether they come from carbohydrate, protein, fat, or alcohol. Plain and simple, if you eat more than you burn, you gain weight, and if you burn more than you eat, you lose weight.

The reason people with diabetes must pay such careful attention to calorie intake is that body fat interferes with insulin's action, causing or exacerbating insulin resistance. Each person's daily calorie needs are unique and are based on factors such as height, current weight, ideal weight, metabolism, and physical activity level. As was the case in determining appropriate carbohydrate intake, it is best to seek the guidance of a registered dietitian to help you figure out how many calories you should aim to consume each day.

Counting calories can be done similarly to counting carbs: You can check the label on packaged foods for calorie content per serving, and you can look up the calorie content of unlabeled foods either on the government's free online nutrient database (see "No Label? No Problem" on page 80) or in a store-bought nutrient guide.

To lose excess body fat, you must burn more calories than you take in. Increasing your physical activity will help to create a calorie deficit. But exercise alone, with no change in caloric intake, rarely results in significant, sustainable weight loss. Most often, a combination of increased calorie expenditure and a modestly reduced calorie intake leads to the greatest weight loss over the long-term.

To meet the reasonable goal of losing one pound of fat per week, you will need to create a 3,500-calorie deficit each week. Adding 30 minutes of exercise most days will get you about halfway there. To make it the rest of the way, you will need to reduce your calorie intake. Cutting just 250 to 300 calories from your daily intake should get the job done.

If adding up the calories in everything you eat doesn't sound practical, don't worry. You can certainly cut your calorie intake just by paying more attention to your diet and using the commonsense techniques that follow. In fact, the reason most commercial diets produce weight loss is simply that they force dieters to think about and plan their daily food intake instead of just eating whatever they feel like eating!

# Trusted Calorie-Cutting Techniques
What follows are 15 ways to make calorie cutting easier and more successful.

### 1. Announce your intentions.
Writing down your goals and putting them on prominent display on your refrigerator or bathroom mirror will help refresh your commitment every day. Share your goals with family members and friends whom you trust to give you encouragement and support. Make your

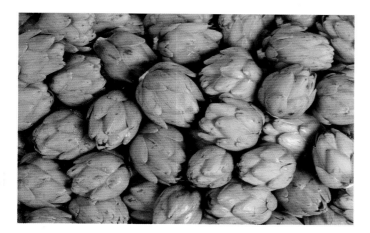

goals specific and realistic: frame your intention as "cut 250 calories a day" and/or "stop snacking after dinner" rather than "eat less."

## 2. Control your blood sugar.

If your blood sugar is out of control, you'll find it harder to control your food intake. If you have high blood sugar levels, your appetite will tend to increase, while lower blood sugar levels require treatment with extra calories.

You're probably wondering how you can control your blood sugar if you don't yet have your eating under control. If this is the case, talk to your doctor about beginning, increasing, or adding diabetes medication to get your blood sugar into a range that will allow you to get your eating under control. In time, as your weight comes down, you will probably be able to cut back on the medication. Likewise, if your current medication

program is causing hypoglycemia more than once or twice a week, talk with your doctor about reducing your dose or switching to a different drug. Hypoglycemia requires immediate calorie intake in the form of rapid-acting carbs and often causes a nearly insatiable appetite, so eliminating the lows can erase the need for those hundreds of extra calories each week.

## 3. Keep a food diary.

Studies show that when most people estimate their food intake, they underestimate it dramatically. One way to be aware of your food intake is to start a food diary. For two weeks, write down precisely what, when, and how much you take in. Be specific—a "salad" might be loaded with vegetables and use light dressing, or it might include chicken strips, cheese, croutons, and full-fat dressing. Keep track of the context as well: where you were, what you were doing, and how you were feeling when you ate. After two weeks, look back over the details. You'll start to see patterns emerging that provide insight into your eating habits. Continue to track as you implement new food strategies. Even after you've attained your goal weight, keeping a food diary will help you maintain your weight loss over the long term.

### 4. Establish a pattern.

One temptation when you're trying to lose weight is to skip meals altogether. However, this tends to cause cravings and intense hunger late in the day, which usually leads to uncontrolled snacking and poor food choices. Having three substantial, evenly spaced meals at roughly the same times each day helps the body to regulate its appetite according to your schedule.

### 5. Opt for less fat.

Fat is much more calorie dense than carbohydrate, protein, or even alcohol. Every gram of fat contains nine calories, whereas a gram of alcohol contains seven and a gram of carbohydrate or protein contains just four. By choosing a low-fat food in place of a high-fat food of equal size, you are likely to eliminate many calories. For example, a four-ounce serving of low-fat frozen yogurt contains about 100 calories, while four ounces of ice cream contain about 150. Although the portions are the same, one has more carbohydrate, the other more fat. However, don't get the idea that something will help you lose weight just because it is low in fat. If it contains carbohydrate, protein, or alcohol, it still has calories, and it can still cause weight

## Small and Frequent Wins the Race

For people who have type 2 diabetes, eating several small meals per day actually tends to produce better blood sugar control than having just three large meals. The only exceptions are the people who take insulin at each meal. For them, giving the insulin time to finish working before eating again produces the best blood sugar control, so they tend to do better with just the three large meals.

gain if eaten in large quantities. (Some low-fat versions even contain *more* calories than their full-fat counterparts, so check labels carefully!)

To help trim fat from your diet:

- Select low-fat snacks. Instead of chips, nuts, cookies, and chocolate, choose low-fat popcorn, low-fat or nonfat yogurt, or fresh fruits and vegetables.
- Eat out less. Food prepared at a restaurant, whether that's a quality sit-down establishment, a fast-food outlet, or a take-out joint, tends to contain a great deal more fat than food that is prepared at home.
- Switch to skim milk. Whole and even two-percent milk contain a great deal more fat. Opt for reduced-fat varieties

90

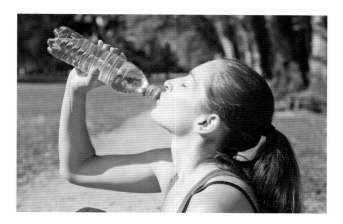

"volume," so they tend to fill you up and curb your appetite, making it easier to skip second helpings. Vegetables are rich in vitamins and minerals we all need for good health, as well.

Get creative. Sample vegetables you've never tried before. Try different low-fat cooking methods, such as steaming, grilling, or stir-frying. Use herbs and spices to enrich flavors. Use seasonal vegetables to make frittatas, risotto, pilafs, or clear soups, or try layering them on sandwiches.

of other dairy products, as well.

- Choose lean cuts of meat. The more "marbling" throughout a cut of beef, the more fat it contains. White-meat poultry and seafood tend to be lower in fat than fowl, dark-meat poultry, beef, and pork. Also, remove the skin prior to eating fowl or poultry.

## 6. Add vegetables.

Meat tends to be high in calories, and starch tends to drive up blood sugar. Vegetables, on the other hand, are typically low in calories and have low GI scores. When you eye your plate, vegetables should take up about half of it, with meat and starches given smaller portions.

Making leafy and crunchy vegetables (fresh or cooked) a more substantial part of every meal helps increase the fiber content of your diet. Because most vegetables are low on the GI chart, they provide slow-burning fuel. They have

## 7. Pay attention to portion sizes.

Even if you make healthy food choices, you can undermine your weight-loss efforts with oversize portions. Sometimes, the serving size listed on a food label doesn't match what we actually eat. Invest in a set of measuring cups and spoons and a basic food scale, and test your ability to "eyeball" portions from time to time.

The typical portion size of many foods has increased dramatically over the past several decades. Today's 20-ounce soda used to be only 8 ounces. The 30-gram bagel has been supplanted by a monstrous 70-gram one. Even movie-theater popcorn has busted its own beltline: A "large" popcorn from the '60s is smaller than a "small" popcorn at most theaters today.

Reducing portion sizes across-the-board has worked for many dieters. Try eating 25 percent or 50 percent less of everything than you're used to having—main courses, side dishes, desserts, beverages. Simply paying attention to your portion sizes may be all it takes to cut down significantly on your calorie intake!

One trick that helps some people to eat less is to use smaller plates and bowls for serving meals. A portion of food that is served on a small plate seems larger than the same portion presented on a large plate.

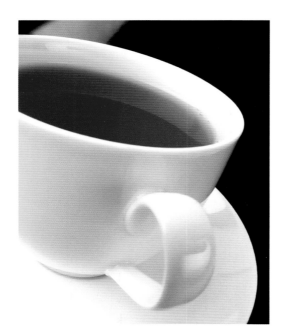

Restaurants are notorious for serving huge portions. So when you eat out, consider ordering child-size portions or asking that half your serving be placed in a doggie bag before it reaches your table. And steer clear of "all you can eat" buffets!

**8. Take your time.**
It can take 30 to 60 minutes for the "full" sensation to register, even after a substantial meal. So slow down. Chew each mouthful thoroughly, and put your fork down between bites. And after finishing your usual portion, get up from the table and do something else: Clear and clean the dishes, take a walk, read your mail, etc. By the time you're done, the feeling of fullness should be setting in, and you will have kept yourself from eating more than you need.

**9. Cut down on snacks.**
If you eat three substantial meals, consider eliminating snacks. If you eat smaller meals that are more than four hours apart, it is reasonable to have a modest snack between those meals. If you do snack, though, be sure to measure out what you are going to eat or consider buying or making single servings (but be sure to eat just one serving); don't eat directly from a full-size bag, package, or container.

### 10. Drink plenty of water.

The recommended water intake per day is about two quarts (eight cups). Research has even shown that your basal metabolic rate (the amount of calories your body burns at rest) may increase up to 30 percent when you start drinking enough water. Thirst is also often mistaken for hunger, so before you snack, drink a glass of water first to see if the feeling of hunger passes. If you don't like plain water, try adding a twist of lemon or lime or a small splash of juice. Decaffeinated and unsweetened tea and coffee, calorie-free drinks, and seltzer also count toward your eight cups a day.

### 11. Avoid "cheap" calories.

It's amazing how many calories we take in without realizing it. Sugary beverages are a good example. A single can of regular soda contains 130 to 180 calories; a can of diet soda usually contains none. Choose sugar-free beverages instead. Sauces, dressings, and gravies are another source of cheap calories. A healthy 100-calorie salad can easily become a 400- to 500-calorie monster when doused in Caesar dressing. Use toppings in moderation, and skip the fat-filled, cream-based varieties.

### 12. Cut down on alcohol.

Like fat, alcohol is very dense in calories. Alcohol contains seven calories per gram, and that's not counting the calories from the carbohydrates that accompany the alcohol in beer, wine, and mixed drinks. Alcohol consumption also interferes with the body's burning of excess fat for fuel. Because alcohol is a toxin the body wants to get rid of as quickly as possible, the body holds off using stored fat for fuel and instead burns the alcohol for fuel. So if you're serious about losing weight and gaining control of your blood sugar, opt for seltzer or diet soda rather than alcoholic beverages most or all of the time.

### 13. Prepare to be hungry sometimes.

There will be times when you'll want to eat when you shouldn't. Remember, however, that you *are* stronger and smarter than your appetite. These strategies may help you handle cravings:

- Since many food cravings are situational rather than physical, try slowly counting to 30 when a craving strikes. It will usually subside.
- When a craving hits, visualize yourself thinner and more fit. Then decide which will make you feel better: looking and feeling that way or eating the food you're craving.
- Engage in a healthy or neutral substitute habit when a craving occurs: Make and drink a cup of unsweetened tea, chew sugarless gum, take a short walk, text a friend,

play a computer game, surf the Web, meditate, etc.

- If you tend to get cravings in certain situations, change your routine. Do something other than watching TV in the evening. Stay out of the kitchen unless you're preparing or eating a meal. Don't allow food in the car.

## 14. Rule out—or treat—other health problems.

Controlling your eating patterns is not always easy. The last thing you need is a secondary health condition that interferes with your efforts. Compulsive eating disorders, for example, occur in nearly half of all overweight people. Binge eating may have a physical or psychological basis that can be treated with therapy and/or medication. Symptoms include:

- eating large quantities of high-calorie foods
- eating secretively
- frequent weight fluctuations of more than ten pounds
- feeling depressed after eating
- feeling that you cannot control your eating

Without realizing it, many people use food for comfort or distraction. Some people are psychologically addicted to food, and they use it as a way of self-medicating an underlying psychological problem. If you habitually use food to make yourself feel better, talk to a therapist who specializes in eating disorders.

Depression is another medical disorder common among people with diabetes. Depression can lead to unhealthy eating patterns. Symptoms include:

- frequent feelings of sadness or dread of the future
- loss of interest or pleasure in daily activities
- crying spells
- fatigue
- sleeping too much or too little
- loss of appetite or overeating
- unusual irritability
- difficulty thinking, concentrating, remembering details making decisions
- feelings of worthlessness or guilt or dwelling on negative thoughts
- suicidal thoughts (if you experience these, seek immediate medical attention)

Talk to your doctor if you experience these or similar symptoms. Talk/behavioral therapy and/or medication can be used quite successfully to treat depression.

Hypothyroidism ("underactive thyroid") is also very common among people who have had diabetes for many years. Thyroid hormone plays a major role in regulating metabolism, so hypothyroidism

can make weight loss very difficult.
Symptoms of hypothyroidism include:

- feeling sluggish
- decreased appetite
- slowed reflexes
- weight gain
- dry skin
- thinning hair
- constipation
- inability to tolerate cold
- impaired memory

Medications for treating hypothyroidism can reverse these symptoms and help restore metabolism to a normal level.

If you suspect that you may have a secondary health condition that is interfering with your ability to lose excess body fat, consult your doctor.

**15. Discuss medication with your doctor.**
A number of diabetes medications have been shown to also curb hunger and help people with type 2 to eat less. Metformin reduces the amount of sugar released by the liver, but it can also cause mild stomach upset and loss of appetite. The noninsulin injectable drugs exenatide (Byetta) and liraglutide (Victoza) improve the ability of the pancreas to produce insulin and slows the rate at which food moves from the stomach into the intestines, which triggers a strong feeling of fullness soon after you start eating. Pramlintide (Symlin), another injectable that slows stomach emptying, also stimulates the satiety (fullness) center of the brain, helping to reduce food cravings. Ask your doctor if any of these medications is appropriate for you.

# Exercise for Glucose Control

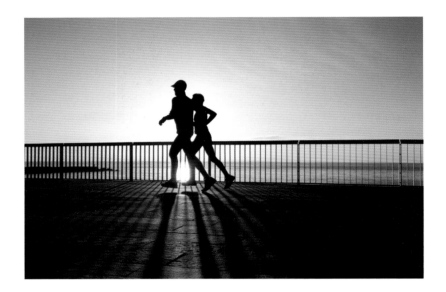

You may not think of a brisk walk, a game of tennis, or an hour spent cleaning your house or yard as medicine for treating your diabetes, but it is. In fact, getting physical will not only help you better manage your diabetes, it will help treat, delay, or even prevent many of the long-term complications associated with the disease.

As discussed in Chapter 2, people with diabetes—whether type 1 or type 2—are at high risk for heart disease, high blood pressure, infection, elevated cholesterol, depression, and increased stress. Physical activity is a proven way to combat all of these conditions. It also burns extra calories—an important added benefit for those who need to lose weight. And working the muscles can make any body—but especially a body with type 2 diabetes—use insulin more efficiently.

Yet research suggests that your current relationship with physical activity may be intimately linked with the form of diabetes you have. According to *The Physician and Sportsmedicine*, a respected medical journal, those who have type 1 diabetes often want to exercise but in certain situations should not, while those who have type 2 diabetes almost always should exercise but often don't want to.

In other words, both groups face challenges when it comes to physical activity. To ensure that exercise doesn't cause more harm than good, those with type 1 (and those with type 2 who use insulin or other medications that can cause hypoglycemia) must take certain precautions and will likely need to do some experimenting to determine how best to juggle activity with medication doses and food intake. Those who have

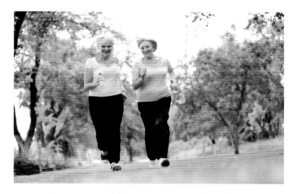

type 2, meanwhile, may need to find creative ways to add movement to their days to overcome a mental resistance to being more physically active.

One thing is clear, however: The benefits of getting physical are worth the effort, whether you have type 1 or type 2. So work with your diabetes care team to create a personalized exercise program that suits your needs, based on the form of diabetes you have, the type of medication(s) you use, whether you have any complications that may affect your choice of physical activity, and whether weight loss is a goal. The information in this chapter can help guide your planning and get you moving toward a more active life.

## Exercise and Type 1

If you have type 1 diabetes, timing is everything when it comes to exercise. Physical activity lowers blood sugar—the longer and more vigorous the workout, the lower blood sugar can drop—so taking steps to make sure the time is right to exercise will help you avoid hypoglycemia.

Indeed, as long as your blood sugar is under control and complications don't limit your mobility or tolerance for exercise, there's no need to sit on the bench. Just follow some simple rules.

1. Avoid vigorous activity if your fasting glucose is above 250 mg/dl and you test positive for ketones.
2. Exercise with caution if your fasting glucose is above 300 mg/dl in the absence of ketosis.
3. Consume carbs before exercising if your glucose level is below 100 mg/dl.
4. Monitor blood sugar before, during, and after exercise. Comparing the results will provide important information about how exercise affects your insulin needs. Based on how your blood sugar changes after a workout, your doctor or diabetes educator will recommend necessary changes to your insulin dose and provide advice about whether you need to consume carbs before exercising. Since you will probably respond differently to a 30-minute swim than a 60-minute walk, be sure to do before-and-after testing for all the different activities you participate in.
5. Keep glucose tablets or another carb source handy in case you become hypoglycemic.

You'll find information on making food and insulin adjustments for exercise at the end of this chapter.

## Incorporating Activity

This doesn't mean you should run out and get a gym membership—especially if you wouldn't use it. Instead, take steps to incorporate more movement in your daily life. Especially if you've been a couch potato of late, those first steps toward becoming more active don't even have to look like exercise in the traditional sense.

Being physically active every day is as much a state of mind as it is a state of being. It means taking every opportunity you can to move more. For many people with blood sugar problems, the simple act of walking more may be enough to start setting things right. To increase

### Stroll Your Way to Success

For a 200-pound person, walking at a slow pace burns about 300 calories per hour. While you're enjoying your favorite television shows, walk on a treadmill or even walk in place as you watch, and you'll see yourself get smaller!

motivation, a pedometer can work wonders. This small device clips onto your waistband and tracks the number of times your hips shift position each day. It counts every time you get up, sit down, turn, jump, and step. It also reminds you that movement is good. Research has shown that people who wear pedometers and check them periodically throughout the day are motivated to walk and move more.

You should be able to find a basic pedometer for under $25. It need not track anything other than the number of steps you take in a day. At the start, wear the pedometer around for a couple of days without changing your normal routine, just to see how many steps you currently average per day. Then aim to add a couple thousand more, and work toward meeting that goal. If you can work your way up to 10,000 steps or more per day, you will almost certainly be burning enough calories to improve your sensitivity to insulin.

## Adding in Movement

Here are some ways to add movement to the course of your daily life:

- Use a cordless or mobile phone. Get in the habit of walking while you talk.
- When you go shopping, park further away from the store's entrance.
- Take the stairs instead of elevators

and escalators, particularly when going only one or two levels.

- At airports, if you're using one of the moving walkways, walk instead of standing still.
- At work, if you need to talk to a colleague on the other side of the building, walk instead of calling or e-mailing.
- If you have a dog, volunteer to be the person who walks it.
- Don't just sit in front of the TV. Hide the TV remote and get up to change channels. Buy a treadmill, stair-stepper, or small elliptical machine, and use it while you watch TV.
- Do your own yard work.
- Do your own housework.

## Develop an Exercise Routine

Once you begin adding more movement into your daily routine, the next step—establishing an exercise routine—will come much easier. Because even though moving more throughout your day can do a lot for you, it can't do everything. To improve your cardiovascular (heart and blood vessel) fitness and make a serious attempt at weight loss, you will need to perform physical activities that are a bit more challenging. You will need to exercise.

To create an exercise routine for yourself, you first need to select a suitable physical activity. To qualify as exercise, an activity needs to engage large muscles in repetitive movement and raise your heart rate and breathing for an extended period of time. Since you are looking to incorporate it into your daily routine, the exercise activity you choose should also be something that you enjoy, that you have easy access to, and that is safe and reasonable for you to perform given your current health, abilities, and schedule. Your selection will also need approval

## Tag Up

If you have type 1 diabetes or you have type 2 but take insulin or another medication that puts you at risk for hypoglycemia, play it safe: Whenever you exercise, wear a bracelet, necklace, or shoe tag identifying yourself as a person with diabetes.

from your physician, especially if you haven't been active recently.

Besides deciding on a type of exercise, you also need to consider when you will exercise, how often, for how long, and how intensely. If you have an exercise physiologist on your diabetes care team, you can work together to devise an effective, challenging, and safe exercise program that evolves as your fitness increases; the information in this chapter can facilitate your discussions. If you don't have access to such a professional, you can use the ideas that follow to design your own exercise program.

## Add Variety

As you build an exercise program, think in terms of variety. You want to build a program with different types of exercise activities. That way, you won't only exercise the same muscles and joints. Having several potential activities to choose from can also keep you from getting bored and cutting your exercise time short.

Think about the weather—don't rely on activities that can only be performed in good weather. In addition, incorporate some activities that you can do at home, so that you're not reliant on a working car to exercise.

## Levels of Impact

To exercise safely, keep your current level of health in mind. For example, those who have problems in their lower extremities would want to incorporate non-weight-bearing exercises such as stationary cycling, water exercise, and upper-body weight lifting. This includes anyone with very poor circulation or loss of nerve sensation in the legs or feet, as well as those with injuries, infections, or problems with balance.

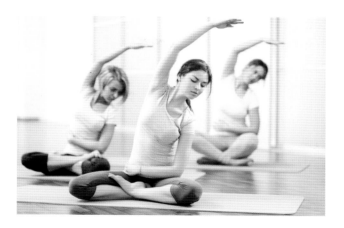

Low-impact aerobic exercises work well for those who haven't exercised regularly in some time. These are activities that don't involve a lot of jumping, pounding, or hitting anything with a lot of force, which can damage muscles, bones, and joints. If your fitness level allows, however, you can include various court sports (tennis, basketball, racquetball, or squash, for example) as well as higher-impact activities (such as running, jumping rope, boxing, or martial arts) that you think you might enjoy. Weight lifting (strength training) also has its place in an exercise program and will be discussed in detail a bit later.

## Frequency

Exercise really does act like medicine for people with diabetes in that it changes the way the body uses insulin. While it's okay to take a day off from exercise every once in a while, it's best to get a daily dose of this medication. In fact, one study of people who successfully maintained long-term weight loss found that they had one important quality in common: They all exercised for about one hour per day.

If you're new to exercise, start with just a few days per week. Increase the amount of exercise you do gradually, over time. Studies show that it takes at least 150 minutes of aerobic exercise per week to attain significant health benefits, including better blood sugar control, reduction of heart disease risk, and weight maintenance. The American Diabetes Association recommends spreading your weekly workout quota over at least three days, while not going more than two consecutive days without exercise.

# A Question of Timing

When you're choosing a time of day to exercise, there are certain factors to keep in mind. Choose a time of day that works well with your schedule and lifestyle, and one that's sustainable. If you hate mornings, don't undercut your long-term success by pledging to get up early each day to exercise.

Exercising at about the same time each day is best for improving blood sugar control and for sticking with an exercise program long-term. Because exercise can make your muscles more sensitive to insulin for several hours following the activity, exercising at the same time each day can help prevent unexpected peaks and valleys in your blood sugar levels. But if you need to vary the timing of your workouts because of other commitments, that's perfectly fine; just be prepared to make adjustments to your insulin or medication as needed.

If possible, you may want to take advantage of the immediate blood-sugar-lowering effect of exercise and do it soon after eating a meal. This especially benefits those who take insulin at each meal and want to lose weight, because they can cut back on their mealtime insulin dose and not have to worry about eating extra food just before exercising to ward off hypoglycemia. However, if you've been diagnosed with heart disease, it is best to wait a couple hours after a meal before exercising, as a weak heart may be overstressed when exercise is performed too soon after eating.

# Intensity

Forget "no pain, no gain." Pain means you're overdoing it or doing something improperly. Exercise should feel *good*. If it doesn't, ease up.

Maintaining moderate intensity while exercising will help you get the most out of a workout without quitting too early. Your goal should be to get your heart beating at 50 to 70 percent of its maximal rate (as measured by beats per minute)

You can take your pulse either at your wrist or, if you don't press too hard, on the side of your Adam's apple.

| Your Age | Ten-Second Target Heart-Rate Range During Exercise |
|----------|------------------------------------------------------|
| 20–29 | 20–26 |
| 30–39 | 19–25 |
| 40–49 | 18–23 |
| 50–59 | 17–22 |
| 60–69 | 16–21 |
| 70–79 | 15–19 |
| 80+ | 14–18 |

Check your pulse as you continue the activity, if possible; otherwise, stop only long enough to count the heartbeats. Counting your pulse for ten seconds will let you know if you are above, below, or within what is called your target heart-rate range during exercise. (Note that these ranges apply only to those who are *not* taking any medication that limits heart rate, such as beta blockers for high blood pressure; if you take any such medication, ask your doctor or exercise physiologist what your target range should be.) If your heart rate during exercise is above the range listed in the table below, slow down. If it is below, speed up a bit. Keep in mind that even if you maintain the same intensity, your heart rate may increase during the course of a workout as you begin to fatigue, so check your pulse every five or ten minutes throughout your workout to ensure you're still in your target range.

If you're having difficulty carrying on a light conversation, you're working too hard. What could be simpler?

## Start Slowly and Cool Down

If you have not exercised for many years (or ever), it is fine to start out at an easy pace for just a few minutes at a time and then gradually build up the length of your exercise sessions by adding one minute each time you exercise. You should aim to reach at least 30 minutes of continuous exercise. If you can go longer and you want to lose weight a little bit quicker, gradually build up to one 60-minute exercise session or two 30-minute exercise sessions each day.

Once you have reached the desired workout length, start to slowly increase your speed or intensity. This will keep you

Another option for tracking your intensity—the talk test—is very unscientific but practical all the same. It relies on this simple guideline: If you're breathing hard but can keep up a casual conversation while exercising, you're probably doing fine. If you can sing, you probably need to push yourself harder.

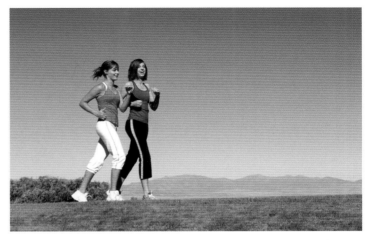

## The Buddy System

You don't have to make these lifestyle changes by yourself. Get support from a spouse, partner, friends, even your children.

- Sign up for a fitness class, or set up a regular workout schedule, with a buddy. This is one case where peer pressure may be a good thing, since you're less likely to blow off a workout if it means letting down a friend.
- Take a dancing class.
- Go on bike rides as a family.
- Instead of meeting friends at a restaurant for a meal, propose a trip to a park, a museum, or an arboretum: someplace where you can walk and talk instead of just sitting.
- Go bowling or play miniature golf instead of going out to movies or shows.

within your target range as your fitness level improves, and it will keep your workouts challenging and stimulating. Your 30 to 60 minutes of exercise per day should include a few minutes of warm-up and cool-down time spent in a slow, easy version of your chosen exercise. If you plan to walk briskly for exercise, for example, start and finish your workout with three to five minutes of casual walking. This allows your heart rate to adjust gradually and safely as you begin and end your workout.

## Jump-Start Your Metabolism

You can burn plenty of additional calories each day by exercising and increasing your overall level of physical activity. But we're going to let you in on a little secret: There's a way you can burn extra calories when you're not lifting a finger. It involves something called your basal metabolic rate.

Your basal metabolic rate refers to the calories your body burns just to keep your heart beating, lungs breathing, eyes blinking...in other words, just to keep you alive. This calorie expenditure is like the interest you earn on a bank account: It's essentially something you get for doing nothing but being there.

Fat is metabolically stagnant. In other words, fat cells require virtually no calories to stay alive. Muscle, on the other hand, is very active metabolically. Muscle cells chew through a lot of calories even when they aren't moving. The more muscle you have, the higher your basal metabolism and the more calories your body burns all the time—even when you're resting. Adding muscle is like turning a savings account that pays 3 percent interest into a high-yield account that earns 8 percent.

Cardiovascular, or aerobic, exercise—like walking or swimming—will tone your muscles, strengthen your heart, improve blood flow throughout your body, and help improve your blood sugar levels. But it won't necessarily do much to make your muscles bigger (if you're a man) or denser (if you're a woman). Adding muscle requires strength training, such as weight lifting. Strength training involves moderate to high exertion for short periods of time. When a muscle is worked to near (but not quite) exhaustion, the muscle becomes stronger and more efficient. Stronger and more efficient muscles burn more calories every minute of the day, whether you are actively working them or not, and they can help you achieve your weight loss goals more quickly.

## Low-Impact Activities

Swimming
Cycling
"Power walking"
Hiking
Rowing
Stair climbing
Using an elliptical trainer
Dancing

If your diabetes care team includes an exercise physiologist, he or she can work with you to design and implement a strength-training routine to suit your needs and abilities. If you have access to a health club, ask a member of the fitness staff to demonstrate how to use the various machines properly. If you plan to lift weights on your own, you can use ordinary household objects for weights: unopened food cans, plastic jugs filled with water or sand, rocks, rolls of coins, or anything else that is small, dense, and easy to grip. Ask your doctor or certified diabetes educator or check online for some basic strengthening exercises you can perform without machines. You'll find information on designing a strengthening routine below.

As with any form of exercise, when you start lifting weights, it is best to start very slow and easy; otherwise, you could wind up very sore and discouraged afterward. As time goes on, gradually increase the number of repetitions (reps) you do of each weight-lifting exercise. Increase the amount of weight you use as well. Don't get discouraged if you reach a plateau and find it difficult to increase the weight or do additional reps; everyone hits plateaus at some points. Just work on perfecting your technique.

| Medications that Can Cause Hypoglycemia | Medications that Do Not Cause Hypoglycemia |
|---|---|
| • **Insulin** (all forms)<br>• **Sulfonylureas** (glipizide, glyburide)<br>• **Meglitinides** (Prandin, Starlix)<br>• **Combination Medications** that contain any of the above | • **Metformin** (Glucophage)<br>• **Acarbose** (Precose)<br>• **Thiazoladinediones** (Actos, Avandia)<br>• **DPP4 Inhibitors** (Januvia)<br>• **Incretin Mimetics** (Byetta, Symlin) |

You will progress faster and/or further or reach a plateau sooner on some exercises than you do on others. It helps to track your weight-lifting progress by keeping a simple log. For each exercise in your routine, write down the date, the weight you used, and the number of sets and reps you were able to perform before you no longer had the strength to lift the weight or do the exercise properly. The next time you do the exercise, check this record to see how far you got with it the last time, and try to take it a step further.

Here are some pointers to help make your weight-lifting workouts safer and more effective:

1. Warm up before lifting. Walk or ride a stationary bike for a few minutes before you begin a round of weight-lifting, and mimic each exercise (minus the weight) before performing it.

2. Lift in the proper order. Start with exercises that work the big muscles in the chest, back, thighs, and shoulders, and end with lifts that train the smaller muscles of the arms and lower legs. When going through your lifting routine, try to alternate between exercises that work your arms and shoulders, those that strengthen your abdomen and lower back, and those that focus on your buttocks and legs.

3. Never hold your breath when lifting weight. This can cause a dangerous rise in blood pressure. Blow air out when you raise the weight, and inhale as you lower it.

4. Skip a day between weight-lifting workouts to give muscles time to recover and become stronger.

5. When increasing weight, do so in very small increments. For example, go from

106

lifting five pounds to six or seven (maybe 7.5) pounds.

6. Do not proceed until your technique is perfect. Be sure you can maintain the proper form for every single rep before you increase the weight or the number of reps. If you struggle with the last couple of reps, stay where you are until you can do them all properly.

7. Lift and lower weight using slow, controlled movements. Slow lifts produce the best results.

## Adjust for Physical Activity

Sometimes, the truth hurts. One truism facing people with diabetes is this: The more insulin you take—or the more insulin your body makes—the harder it is to burn fat and lose weight. But the opposite is also true: The less insulin you take (or make), the easier it is for your body to shed fat. That's why it's so important to take advantage of any opportunity that allows you to cut back on your insulin levels without harming blood sugar control.

Physical activity creates such an opportunity. Because physical activity makes your insulin work far more effectively, you don't need as much of it. In fact, if you inject insulin or use a medication that stimulates your pancreas to make more insulin, and you *don't* reduce your medication dose to account for physical activity, you could wind up with hypoglycemia.

If you do not use a medication that can cause hypoglycemia, you don't need to worry about snacking, reducing your medication dose, or doing anything else before or during your workouts to adjust for exercise.

If you do use insulin or a drug that increases your body's insulin production, you will need to make some commonsense adjustments that will help you prevent low blood sugar and lose weight faster; they are discussed below. Just be sure to check with your diabetes care team before making any of your own dosage adjustments.

If you take rapid-acting insulin at mealtimes or use a pre-mixed formulation that contains rapid-acting insulin, it is a good idea to reduce your insulin dose at the meal prior to your physical activity. Work with your diabetes care team to determine doses that work for you. Also, you should be prepared for the possibility of a delayed blood sugar drop, particularly after a long or very intense workout. There are two reasons such a drop can occur. The muscle cells' enhanced sensitivity to insulin, which normally occurs after activity, is prolonged when the exercise itself is prolonged. And the muscle cells need to replenish their own energy stores following such exhaustive exercise. If you tend to experience a drop in blood sugar several hours after heavy exercise, you can prevent it by lowering your long-acting and rapid-acting insulin by 25 percent following the workout or by having an extra snack prior to the time the drop in blood sugar tends to occur. Ideally, the snack should contain slowly digesting carbohydrates, such as whole fruit, milk, yogurt, or peanut butter.

If you take insulin or a medication that can cause hypoglycemia, there are certain situations in which you will need to consume extra food to prevent hypoglycemia. One example is when you will be exercising before or between meals. The size of the snack you'll need will depend on the duration and intensity of your workout. The harder and longer your muscles will be working, the more carbohydrate you will need to maintain

## Don't Skimp on Equipment

Good-quality exercise equipment pays for itself in the form of better protection against injuries. In particular, good athletic shoes are a must for nearly all types of cardiovascular, or aerobic, exercise. When exercising, wear shoes with air or gel midsoles (the shock-absorbing pads between the soles and feet) and a generous toe box. Always wear socks to keep your feet dry. Making sure that the shoes you plan to purchase— or the ones you already own—fit properly will save you a lot of trouble later on.

your blood sugar level. The amount is also based on your body size: The bigger you are, the more fuel you will burn while exercising and the more carbohydrate you will need.

To confirm that you have chosen the optimal size and frequency for your snacks, test your blood sugar before and after the activity. If it has held steady, you chose the right amount. If it has gone up, you will need to cut back on the grams of carbohydrate you eat before each hour of exercise next time. And if your blood sugar has dropped, you will need to eat more carbohydrate before each hour of

# A Few Words of Caution

Although all diabetes patients should strive to be physically active, some forms of exercise require extra precautions (or may be too risky, period) for people who have any of the following complications. Talk with your diabetes care team about forms of exercise that might cause you health risks because of complications.

## Autonomic Neuropathy

Patients who have this form of nerve damage may not be able to detect symptoms such as sweating and rapid heart rate that signal the onset of exercise-induced hypoglycemia. They also have a high risk for orthostatic hypotension (a drop in blood pressure that can cause dizziness or fainting) during exercise performed while upright, so cycling or swimming may be better choices than walking or running. Beware of exercising in very hot or cold climates, and drink plenty of water.

## Retinopathy

Some types of physical activity increase the risk of a hemorrhage in the eye or a detached retina. Avoid activities that involve a lot of jarring or straining, such as jogging or weight lifting.

## Peripheral Neuropathy

If you can't feel your feet, how will you know if you're pounding the pavement too hard? People with serious loss of sensation in the lower limbs should not overdo weight-bearing exercise. Repetitive, intense pressure on the feet can cause ulcers. You may also fail to realize that you have broken a foot bone. If you have nerve damage that limits feeling in your feet, low-impact exercise, such as swimming, cycling, or rowing, may be the best choice.

exercise or eat more frequently during your exercise session the next time. (Keep track of such information in your exercise log.)

If you take a medication other than insulin that can cause hypoglycemia, it is usually recommended that you take your usual dose for your first couple of exercise sessions and see what happens. If your blood sugar drops below 80 mg/dl during or after exercise, alert your diabetes care team. You may need to reduce or eliminate the medication or switch to a medication that does not cause hypoglycemia. Check with your doctor before you make any medication changes, however.

Despite the precautions you take, hypoglycemia can still occur if you take insulin or a medication that stimulates the release of insulin. So you should always carry a source of simple sugar (such as glucose tablets, a sports drink, juice, or hard candy) and wear a medical alert bracelet or necklace whenever you exercise. Stop the activity and treat the low blood sugar as soon as you suspect it, and take a timeout of at least 15 to 20 minutes to allow the food to be absorbed. Wait until your blood sugar is a minimum of 90 mg/dl before continuing physical activity.

Oddly enough, physical activity can actually increase blood sugar in certain circumstances, particularly at the onset of high-intensity, short-duration exercise.

The cause is a surge of the stress hormone adrenaline. If you detect such an increase, talk with your doctor about ways to offset or prevent it. Although high blood sugar can impair your performance during exercise, it is not necessarily dangerous to exercise when blood sugar levels are moderately elevated. If you experience high blood sugar during exercise, drink plenty of water both during and after your workouts.

If you experience very high blood sugar with exercise, alert your doctor and ask whether you should be checking your urine for ketones, which are acidic byproducts produced when fat is metabolized. It is a good idea to check for ketones if your blood sugar is greater than 300 mg/dl. A positive ketone test could mean that you are deficient in insulin, and in that case, physical activity will probably make your blood sugar go much higher. Do not exercise if your urine contains ketones.

# Relax for Better Blood Sugar

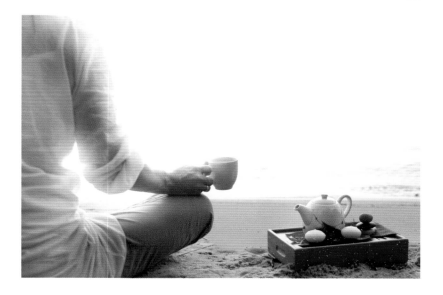

When you feel stressed, your body naturally releases more sugar into your blood. It's the human condition, not the result of diabetes. But if you have diabetes and are trying to improve your blood sugar control, relieving stress should be part of your efforts.

## Your Body Under Stress

Whether the cause of your stress is physical or emotional, your body will have a physical response. Stress causes an adrenaline rush, which increases the heart rate, dilates the pupils, tenses the muscles, causes sweating, stops digestion, and makes the liver release a jolt of sugar into the bloodstream for quick energy. In some scenarios, this stress response is a helpful one. If you're under physical threat, quick energy is a good thing! However, we can have the same response to everyday mental stress, and that's less helpful. You don't want your blood pressure, heart rate, and blood sugar level to rise every time you're stuck in rush hour traffic.

## The Stress Response and Diabetes

For people with diabetes, managing a stress response can be especially important. The stress hormones that cause the liver to secrete extra sugar

into the blood in response to fear, anger, tension, or excitement also increase insulin resistance. For people without diabetes, the stress-induced rise in blood sugar is followed by an increase in insulin secretion, so the blood sugar spike is modest and momentary. For people with diabetes, however, stress can cause blood sugar to rise quickly and stay high for quite a while.

## Reducing Stress

We all have some degree of stress in our lives. You can't cut out stress completely—in fact, since even happy events can cause stress, you wouldn't want to! However, you want to minimize its impact on your life.

Start by figuring out what causes you stress on an everyday basis, whether it's certain people or common situations. Are there ways you can avoid these stressors? If not, how can you reduce their impact on you?

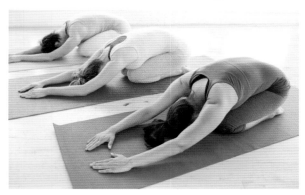

**Minimize interpersonal stress.** Unfortunately, other people can cause us lots of stress, and it's useless to try to change other people. With some people, you might want to minimize contact. With others, it is useful to try to understand why they act the way they do, and don't take their actions too personally.

Even people whose company we enjoy can cause stress. Think carefully about how you want to spend your time and energy, and don't be afraid to say no to other people's requests for your time or energy.

**Talk it out.** Some people benefit from journaling. Just writing a problem down on paper seems to help clarify potential responses or decrease negative emotions. Others prefer to talk things out with a spouse, partner, friend, or therapist. If you're having problems with stress, don't be afraid to seek out a mental health professional. Clinical depression is very common to people with diabetes, and a mental health professional can determine if it might be playing a part.

**Take a break.** Make time for your hobbies. Take a stroll after dinner. Schedule a massage or aromatherapy session. Go to a concert. Take a scenic drive and turn the music on.

> When you can, look for the humorous side of things. When you laugh, your body produces natural painkillers and increases circulation.

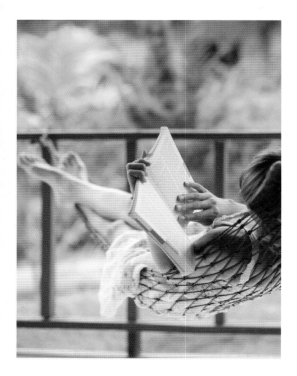

**Take advantage of endorphins.** Spend some time exercising. Hitting baseballs in a batting cage can be a great form of stress relief! Consider taking up the practice of yoga, pilates, tai chi, or some other form of relaxing movement. Virtually every health club, YMCA, and adult education program offers classes that teach such activities. Many hospitals do, as well.

**Get your eight hours of sleep.** When we're sleep deprived, we're likely to become stressed more easily. Fatigue can be a source of physical and emotional stress in its own right.

**Have a plan.** If certain situations always stress you out, have a plan for dealing with them. If you hate waiting in lines, plan ahead for things to do while you wait. Load up your mp3 player with audio books or upbeat music when you need to take a long drive. Write mental scripts for potentially difficult conversations.

**Relax your muscles.** Tighten and release your muscles one group at a time, from face to toes, spending about ten seconds on each muscle group. This forces your muscles to relax. Simply knowing how your muscles feel when you are relaxed will make it easier for you to detect when you're feeling tense in response to stress.

# Take Prescribed Meds

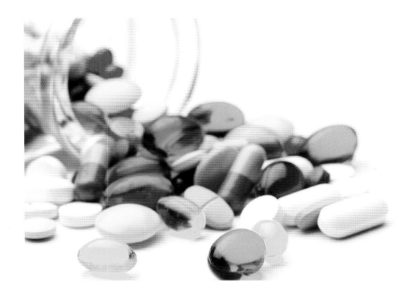

Okay, so perhaps your efforts at treating your type 2 diabetes through dietary changes, exercise, and weight loss weren't enough to get your blood sugar into a safe range. Or perhaps they did help for a few months or even years, but now your blood sugar levels have begun to creep upward again. If you don't do something more to get your disease under control, you may soon begin to feel the effects of your raging blood sugar levels from head to toe.

Fortunately, your doctor can prescribe one or more medications that—when added to your ongoing diet and exercise regimen—can help. (That's right: Drugs for treating diabetes are used *in addition to*, not in place of, lifestyle changes.) Most of the medications that are used to treat type 2 diabetes work by doing one or more of the following:

- decreasing the amount of glucose that the liver releases into the bloodstream
- prompting the pancreas to increase the supply of insulin
- making the body's cells more sensitive to insulin
- reducing the rate at which the body absorbs sugar from food
- controlling appetite and blunting huge glucose spikes following meals

The good news: The majority of these drugs come in the form of a pill. The not-as-good news: Many of them can cause side effects ranging from bothersome to debilitating, although in many cases these effects fade over time or can be relieved by adjusting the dosage of the drug. You will probably have to take whatever drug or combination of drugs your doctor prescribes on an ongoing basis, perhaps even for the rest of your life. But remember: Research shows that controlling blood sugar can postpone or prevent frightening diabetes complications.

# Oral Drugs

The following types of medication act in different ways, but all work toward moving blood sugar levels into a healthier range.

# Biguanides

**Includes: metformin (Fortamet, Glucophage and Glucophage XR, Glumetza, Riomet)**

The single drug in this category is metformin, and it is currently the most frequently prescribed medication for treating type 2 diabetes in the world. Metformin is a multitalented drug. For example, one way that it helps to control blood sugar is by making muscle cells more sensitive to insulin, so they can more easily pull glucose out of your bloodstream.

# Is Metformin Safe?

In a word, yes, though you may have heard that it causes a rare but deadly complication called lactic acidosis. Here's the reality: A predecessor of metformin, known as phenformin, was introduced in the 1950s. Phenformin worked like a charm, but it was banned in the United States in 1977 because some patients who took the drug developed lactic acidosis. Lactic acid is a waste product produced by cells when they burn glucose during hard exercise or other times when oxygen levels in the body are low. When too much lactic acid builds up, muscle pain, erratic heartbeat, rapid breathing, and other problems can result. Lactic acidosis is fatal about 40 percent of the time.

Scientists reconfigured the drug to eliminate the lactic acidosis threat, and Bristol-Myers Squibb introduced the new version, known as metformin, in 1995. Not surprisingly, doubts about the drug linger, and occasional reports arise of lactic acidosis in patients who take metformin. However, according to a commentary published in the July 2004 edition of *Diabetes Care*, an American Diabetes Association journal, virtually all cases of lactic acidosis linked to metformin have been in patients who took overdoses or shouldn't have been taking it in the first place, such as people with kidney disease or an excessive alcohol intake. According to the commentary, when metformin is used as labeled, the increased risk of lactic acidosis is either zero or very close to zero.

But metformin's main role is to get the liver to release less glucose into the bloodstream in the first place. The liver normally stockpiles glucose (which it can make by piecing together fragments of other molecules) and releases it when blood sugar levels dip too low, such as between meals, especially overnight. After all, even when you're dozing, your body still needs glucose; if your glucose dried up, your organs would shut down and even the loudest alarm clock could not wake you.

Normally, the liver slows the release of glucose when there's a lot of insulin in the blood, because that boatload of floating insulin is a sure signal that there's already plenty of sugar in the blood to go around. However, if you have type 2 diabetes, your liver never gets the memo instructing it to stop releasing glucose. It just keeps unloading the sweet stuff into the blood, forcing the pancreas to work overtime to crank out more insulin and making insulin's job of clearing sugar from the blood that much harder. Metformin takes some of the burden off the poor pancreas by fixing the problem with the liver; with less glucose hanging around in the blood, the demand for insulin drops. The medication is typically taken twice a day.

When metformin is used alone, it doesn't cause hypoglycemia. It is also less likely than some other diabetes medications to make you pack on pounds. As a matter of fact, some metformin users even lose weight.

Still, metformin is not free of potential problems. About one-third of patients who take it develop gastrointestinal problems, including upset stomach, gas, diarrhea, and vomiting. (Such unpleasant tummy troubles could have something to do with the weight loss experienced by some metformin users.) Headaches and fatigue may occur, too. The good news is that these side effects usually fade within a few weeks of beginning treatment with metformin. Starting with small doses and gradually building up may also help to forestall unpleasant side effects. Taking metformin with meals can reduce stomach distress, too.

Metformin is often the first medication prescribed to treat type 2 diabetes. But it is not for everyone. The drug should not be used by:

- heavy drinkers
- those with kidney or liver disease
- anyone over 80 years of age, unless tests show that the liver and kidneys are still working hard
- people who have congestive heart failure or any other condition that interferes with circulation
- those with serious asthma or lung disease
- pregnant women
- children

One last word about metformin: It lowers levels of vitamin B12 in 10 to 30 percent of patients. However, taking calcium supplements may offset the drop, since the body needs the mineral to absorb vitamin B12. If metformin has been prescribed for you, ask your doctor if you should take extra calcium, as well.

# Sulfonylureas

**Includes: chlorpropamide (Diabinese), glimepiride (Amaryl), glipizide (Glucotrol and Glucotrol XL), glyburide (Diabeta, Micronase) and micronized glyburide (Glynase)**

Until this class of drugs was introduced in the 1950s, insulin was the only treatment available for people with diabetes. Sulfonylureas work by stimulating the beta cells in the pancreas to release more insulin into the bloodstream. They're usually taken once or twice a day before meals.

The sulfonylureas are usually broken down into older "first generation" pills and newer "second generation" pills. First generation sulfonylureas have fallen out of favor because, in general, the second generation versions are more potent and have fewer side effects. Indeed, the only first-generation sulfonylurea still being used today is chlorpropamide. But the second generation isn't without its faults.

For example, these drugs, like the first-generation sulfonylureas, can cause hypoglycemia. A healthy pancreas is acutely sensitive to glucose levels in the blood, so it only produces as much insulin as the body needs. But sulfonylureas keep the beta cells working all the time, so a steady stream of insulin pours into the blood whether it's needed or not. As a result, blood sugar levels can drop too low, causing hypoglycemia. (This problem is especially common in the elderly and people who have liver or kidney disease.) On the other hand, if the prescribed dose of sulfonylurea is too low, the blood sugar can remain too high and continue to cause damage to the body. The prescribing physician can tinker with the dose to help relieve these problems, however.

Sulfonylureas can also cause weight gain as well as heartburn and other stomach problems. And drinking alcohol while taking certain sulfonylurea drugs may cause nausea, vomiting, and flushed skin.

Finally, sulfonylureas can sometimes lose their ability to control a person's blood sugar levels. Diabetes is a progressive disease, so over time, some of the insulin-producing beta cells in the pancreas will simply die off or slow down production. As beta-cell function decreases, the same amount of a sulfonylurea medication will be less effective at reducing glucose. When this occurs, the patient's doctor may prescribe another sulfonylurea instead or may simply drop the sulfonylurea altogether and switch the patient to another type of diabetes medication.

# Meglitinides
**Includes: nateglinide (Starlix), repaglinide (Prandin)**
These drugs act like sulfonylureas that have had too much caffeine. They are even sometimes referred to as nonsulfonylurea secretagogues because, like sulfonylureas, they trigger the beta cells of the pancreas to "secrete," or release, insulin. The difference is that meglitinides are impatient: They want that insulin released *now*. What's more, while sulfonylureas linger in the body

all day, meglitinides rush in and out quickly. Because of their hyperactive nature, meglitinides play a specific role in managing type 2 diabetes: They are taken immediately before each of a day's three meals to boost insulin production in order to lower the predictable post-meal rise in blood sugar. (And if a meal is skipped, the dose of meglitinide is skipped as well.)

Meglitinides appear to cause hypoglycemia less often than sulfonylureas do, but it's still a possibility, especially if the dose is too high. Meglitinides can also cause weight gain. Other side effects are uncommon but can include backaches, headaches, cold and flu symptoms, chest pain, gastrointestinal problems, joint pain, tingling skin, certain infections, and vomiting.

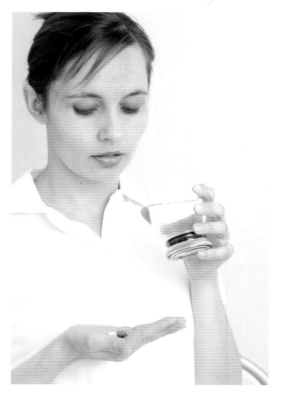

## Thiazolidinediones (Glitazones or TZDs)

**Includes: pioglitazone (Actos), rosiglitazone (Avandia)**

Medications in this group are sometimes referred to as insulin sensitizers, which is a clue to how they work. Remember that in the person with type 2 diabetes, problems begin with the condition known as insulin resistance. The pancreas does its job of releasing insulin, and the insulin tries mightily to usher glucose into muscle and fat cells, but too often, the cells' insulin resistance prevents the hormone from succeeding. As a result, the pancreas must work harder to make more insulin in order for the cells to get the fuel they need. It's as though the cells can't hear insulin molecules knocking until there's a mob of them outside the door.

The glitazones make cells more sensitive to insulin so that they respond to a light tap on the door and allow glucose to enter. Of course, the actual way glitazones work is a bit more complex, but the bottom line is this: These drugs reduce insulin resistance, which helps keep blood sugar levels under control. The insulin-making beta cells of the pancreas, in turn, don't have to work so hard. That means they're less likely to conk out altogether and leave the body dependent on injections of insulin.

While the glitazones increase insulin sensitivity, they do not actually cause the body to make more of the hormone. Therefore, when used alone, glitazones do not cause low blood sugar.

The Food and Drug Administration (FDA) ordered an early version of these drugs, called troglitazone (under the brand name Rezulin), taken off the market in the United States in 2000. The problem: While troglitazone did a spiffy job of controlling blood sugar, in rare cases it caused serious—sometimes fatal—liver damage. The FDA declared that two other similar drugs, rosiglitazone and pioglitazone, were safer to use, although rosiglitazone has been associated with liver abnormalities. If your doctor prescribes one of these two drugs, therefore, he or she will undoubtedly insist on monitoring your liver function through occasional blood tests.

The FDA also recently lifted restrictions on the use of rosiglitazone that it put in place back in 2010. Those restrictions were prompted by a different concern: short-term study results suggesting that the drug caused an increased risk of

heart attack compared to metformin and sulfonylureas. In late 2013, however, the FDA removed most of those restrictions, stating that both a re-evaluation of the original research by outside experts as well as its own review of longer-term study data indicate that rosiglitazone is no more likely to cause a heart attack than the two standard types of diabetes medications. Still, the agency concedes that some "scientific uncertainty" about the cardiovascular safety of rosiglitazone remains. So it's very important that people with type 2 diabetes work very closely with their physicians to determine if rosiglitazone's potential benefits outweigh its risks for them specifically before starting this drug.

As with many diabetes drugs, the glitazones may cause weight gain. Other possible side effects include headache, backache, muscle aches, fatigue, sinus inflammation, and swelling or fluid retention. Furthermore, this class of medication is not recommended for use by anyone who is pregnant. And female patients of childbearing age may need to take extra precautions if they don't want to get pregnant, because the glitazones can lower blood levels of oral contraceptives, making them less effective. Glitazones also appear to increase ovulation in some women, making them more fertile.

## Can Dividing Pills Save You Money?

Maybe. Drug manufacturers often charge the same price for different dosages of the same medication. Patients who pay for their own drugs sometimes ask their doctors to prescribe double doses, which they split in half to save cash. The practice is perfectly safe with certain pills, according to the *Medical Letter on Drugs and Therapeutics,* an independent nonprofit publication for physicians that reviews and evaluates drugs. That includes several widely used diabetes drugs. If your doctor agrees to prescribe a double dose, follow these simple rules:

- Use a pill cutter (available in drugstores) instead of a razor or old butter knife to avoid cutting yourself or ruining part of the pill.
- To maintain even dosing, always take the two halves of a split pill consecutively. Some patients chop up a month's worth of pills all at once, then dump the fragments back in the bottle. But studies show that it's just about impossible to produce evenly cut pill fragments. Pop small fragments for several days in a row, and your blood levels of the drug could drop too low—or vice versa.
- Never split pills without your doctor's consent. Some pills (such as capsules) should not be divided.

Pill splitting may not only be for self-payers, since some insurers have begun to offer lower co-payments to customers who agree to divide their oral medications. Ask your provider about cutting yourself a deal.

## Alpha-Glucosidase Inhibitors (AGIs)

**Includes: acarbose (Precose), miglitol (Glyset)**

Alpha-glucosidase is a type of enzyme that lines the small intestine. Its job is to break down certain forms of sugar— starches, such as bread and potatoes, and sucrose, or table sugar—into glucose molecules small enough to pass into the bloodstream. Alpha-glucosidase inhibitors (AGIs) interfere with these enzymes, delaying the digestion and absorption of these sugars. These medications are taken with the first bite of food to help prevent post-meal sugar spikes. (If a meal is skipped, the dose of the AGI is skipped.)

AGIs are not without their faults, however. Have you ever eaten a bowl of steaming baked beans or other similarly bean-laden dish, then experienced certain uncomfortable and socially embarrassing side effects the next day? The same thing can happen with AGIs. Beans are packed with fiber, which your body can't digest. Like fiber, all the starch that is more slowly digested when you use an AGI eventually makes it to the large intestine, where it becomes fodder for the good bacteria normally living there. The process by which bacteria break down fiber, starch, or any other undigested sugar produces gas. Lots of it. The resulting flatulence, abdominal pain, and diarrhea can be bad enough that some patients plead with their doctors to give them a prescription for some other drug. Some patients find that these problems with the body's food-processing apparatus aren't as severe if they start with a small dose.

AGIs don't cause hypoglycemia, although taking them with certain other diabetic drugs can produce low blood sugar. If hypoglycemia does develop during

## Combining Drugs

Each of the medications discussed in this chapter has something to offer people with type 2 diabetes. But, like a hot dog and mustard, some things work better in combination than they do alone. If you are taking an oral diabetes drug, chances are you will eventually need a second and possibly a third medication to keep your glucose under control. In fact, for every 100 patients with type 2 diabetes who begin taking oral drugs today, 50 will need a second drug to keep their blood sugar under control within three years. In nine years, 75 of those patients will require a combination of pills, according to the August 2005 issue of *Treatment Guidelines from the Medical Letter,* an independently published newsletter for physicians.

The drug metformin may be paired with a sulfonylurea, for example. The rationale for this combination is simple: They complement one another. Metformin reduces the amount of glucose released by the liver into the bloodstream, while the sulfonylurea stimulates the pancreas to increase insulin production, which helps move more glucose out of the bloodstream and into the cells. Together they can be very effective in lowering elevated glucose levels. Indeed, the pairing of these two medications is common enough in diabetes treatment that scientists developed a pill—called Glucovance—that combines them. Other pills that contain two types of diabetes medications are also available.

treatment with one of these drugs, certain sugary foods—the ones affected by AGIs—will not be effective in quickly bringing blood sugar back up to the normal range. Glucose tablets, honey, or fruit juice will still do the trick, however.

If you have had any serious intestinal condition in the past, your doctor probably won't recommend these drugs. Likewise, AGIs are usually considered off-limits for pregnant women.

# Non-Insulin Injectable Drugs

In recent years, scientists have developed some promising new diabetes drugs that do not contain insulin but still must be injected. No, the developers weren't trying to be mean by opting for the injectable form. These drugs simply must be injected in order to bypass the stomach and enter the bloodstream directly. And the tiny needle stick is worth the payoff—better glucose control.

# Incretin Mimetics

**Includes: exenatide (Byetta), Liraglutide (Victoza)**

The Gila monster is a brawny, two-foot-long lizard with a brutal, venomous bite that lives in the desert of the southwestern United States. Why the zoology lesson? Because this scaly critter produces a hormone that may be the key

to better glucose control for some people with type 2 diabetes.

Here's the reason: The Gila monster only eats four times a year—mostly small animals, eggs, and whatever else it can find. The rest of the year, the big lizard survives off fat packed away in its chunky tail and belly. Since it would be pointless, and probably not too healthy, to keep cranking out insulin during those long months between meals, the Gila monster's body evolved the ability to turn off its pancreas. That led researchers to wonder: When a Gila monster finally does sit down to dinner, it needs insulin to process food. How does it turn its pancreas back on?

Scientists eventually discovered a hormone called exendin-4 in the Gila monster's saliva, of all places. (Collecting Gila spit is probably not the highlight of a lab assistant's day.) To be more precise, exendin-4 is an incretin hormone that's produced in the intestines. Humans make incretins, too. When you eat, your gut senses glucose and immediately sends incretins to the pancreas with orders to produce insulin. But in people with type 2 diabetes, the signal from incretins is too weak to stimulate insulin production. Exendin-4, on the other hand, has to be potent enough to arouse a pancreas that's been snoozing for months. The injectable diabetes drug exenatide is a synthetic version of exendin-4 Because exenatide imitates (or "mimes") exendin-4, it's called an incretin mimetic.

Studies show that exenatide keeps blood sugar low not only by stimulating insulin production but also by instructing the pancreas to make less of that other critical hormone, glucagon. As glucagon is suppressed, the liver in turn puts out less glucose. That means less strain on the pancreas. In fact, some research suggests that exenatide even causes the pancreas to make new insulin-producing beta cells in the pancreas.

Exenatide also causes food to pass through your stomach at a more leisurely rate, which slows the typically rapid rise in glucose after a meal. It also means your belly feels full longer, so you eat less. In fact, while most diabetes drugs cause weight gain, exenatide seems to have the opposite effect. In one study, people with type 2 diabetes who took the drug for 30 weeks lost more than six pounds, on average.

So what's the catch? Although it's a powerful drug, exenatide is rather delicate in one sense: It can't tolerate the rough trip through your gastrointestinal system, so it has to be injected just like insulin. Exenatide doses come in prepackaged "pens," similar to the ones used by many diabetes patients who require insulin injections. Exenatide users give themselves two injections per day, before breakfast and dinner. Because most people would rather swallow a pill than stick a needle into their belly or backside, doctors may not prescribe exenatide unless other oral diabetes pills fail to keep a patient's glucose under control.

Exenatide can cause nausea, though it often fades over time. Some other side effects that users have reported include vomiting, diarrhea, the jitters, dizziness, headaches, and upset stomach. Taken alone, exenatide doesn't cause hypoglycemia, but blood sugar may drop too low if the drug is paired with one of the sulfonylureas. People who have kidney disease or serious gastrointestinal problems shouldn't use exenatide. Animal studies show that exenatide may harm fetuses, so women who use the drug and become pregnant may be switched to another medication.

# Amylin Mimetics

**Includes: pramlintide (Symlin)**

Let's get the unwelcome news out of the way first: Like exenatide, pramlintide is an injected drug. Then again, if your doctor prescribes pramlintide, you are

## What about Herbal Therapy?

Walk into any vitamin shop or health food store and you'll find plenty of pills and other products bearing label claims like "maintains healthy sugar" or "boosts insulin." Surf online and you'll find even more "natural" products that sure sound like they would benefit someone with diabetes. These herbs, vitamins, minerals, and other dietary supplements are often (but not always) cheap, and you can take them without a prescription. Should you?

Only if you meet two conditions: If your doctor says it's okay, and if you're a gambler. Dietary supplements are not closely regulated by the Food and Drug Administration (FDA). While new drugs have to undergo extensive testing before hitting the market, dietary supplements are regulated more like food; that is, any company can sell them without having to prove that the products do much of anything.

And that's just the problem. None of the herbs and supplements marketed to people with diabetes has been adequately studied, so you have no way of knowing whether any of them helps control blood sugar. For instance, some supplement sellers claim that high doses of the mineral chromium can reduce insulin resistance. However, the authors of a review in the journal *Diabetes Care* called the evidence for that claim "inconclusive." In fact, the authors examined every study they could find in which natural pills and potions were used to control glucose levels and found that "there is insufficient evidence to actively recommend or discourage use of any particular supplement...."

Ginseng, cinnamon, vitamin E, or any of the other natural pills touted as blood sugar saviors might actually be beneficial. But until more evidence is available, such claims are hard to swallow.

probably already accustomed to pricking and poking yourself, since the medication is used in conjunction with insulin injections. That means it can be used by folks with type 1 diabetes as well as those with type 2.

Pramlintide is a synthetic version of yet another hormone that plays an important role in controlling blood sugar. It turns out that the beta cells in the pancreas hold down two jobs. Not only do they produce insulin, they also make the

# The Latest Drugs for Type 2

In spring 2013, a new kind of oral medication for treating the high blood sugar levels of type 2 diabetes was cleared by the Food & Drug Administration (FDA) for sale in the United States. The drug, manufactured by Johnson & Johnson and called canagliflozin (Invokana), is the first of a new category of diabetes medications called SGLT-2 inhibitors.

Unlike all of the other diabetes medications, SGLT-2 inhibitors target the body's filtration system—the kidneys. All of the blood in the body passes through the kidneys to be cleaned of waste and other undesirable stuff. In folks without diabetes, the kidneys take all the sugar they filter from the blood and shoot it back into the bloodstream through tunnellike proteins, including SGLT-2. In people who have diabetes, however, the kidneys appear to have too many of these tunnels, and even though the blood is overstocked with sugar, the kidneys can't help but send a lot of it back into circulation. The SGLT-2 inhibitors essentially plug up these tunnels, lowering blood sugar levels but without causing hypoglycemia.

Studies suggest canagliflozin, which is taken once daily, is safe and effective at causing significant decreases in A1c levels in people with type 2 diabetes. It also appears to lower the systolic (upper) blood pressure measurement in people with high blood pressure and diabetes.

The drug is not for those with type 1 diabetes or people with type 2 who have ketoacidosis or kidney problems or are under the age of 18. It can cause dehydration as well as urinary tract infections. SGLT-2 inhibitors also tend to increase LDL, the unhealthy form of cholesterol in the blood, and some scientists worry canagliflozin may increase the risk of heart disease, which is bad news for people already at higher risk of heart troubles.

Still, this group of medications appears to show real promise, and more information about their usefulness in helping people with type 2 diabetes is sure to come.

hormone amylin. Beta cells churn out amylin at the same time as insulin when we eat. Like the incretins discussed previously, amylin lowers glucagon levels, so the liver doesn't release unneeded glucose. It also makes the stomach empty into the intestines more slowly after a meal, which prevents glucose spikes.

Unfortunately, if you have type 2 diabetes, your beta cells may be so beat up that you're not producing enough amylin. If you have type 1 diabetes, you probably aren't making the hormone at all. By replacing amylin, therefore, pramlintide helps keep blood sugar levels stable after meals. Some users even lose a few pounds. Your doctor will only add pramlintide to your daily regimen if insulin injections have failed to lower your glucose levels into the safe zone.

Pramlintide is injected just like insulin at mealtimes. But the two hormones don't blend well, so you can't combine the two drugs into one syringe. If you need to take both drugs, you'll still have to inject twice.

Monitoring your blood sugar is a must if you're using pramlintide (as it is if you're injecting insulin); if your blood

sugar is a bit on the low side, a dose of the drug could send it into a freefall and you'll develop severe hypoglycemia. The most common side effect of pramlintide is nausea, followed by loss of appetite, headache, vomiting, stomach pain, fatigue, dizziness, and upset stomach. You might also develop redness, pain, or minor bruising at the spot where you inject pramlintide.

It's also important to talk to your doctor about any other medications you may be taking if he or she prescribes pramlintide. Because it slows down activity in your stomach, pramlintide could alter the effectiveness of some drugs.

## Insulin Therapy

When doctors abandoned the old name "non-insulin-dependent diabetes mellitus" in favor of the sleeker "type 2

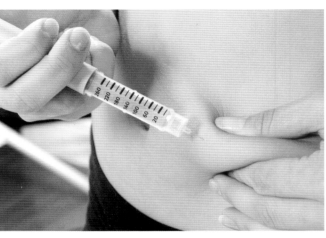

diabetes," they weren't merely opting for a more minimalist, time-saving moniker. Instead, they were acknowledging that, for at least one-quarter of their patients with the condition, the old name is just plain wrong. Although most people with type 2 diabetes have a functioning pancreas when first diagnosed, over time their beta cells may not be able to keep up with demand for insulin, even if oral or noninsulin injectable diabetes drugs are added to diet and exercise therapy.

Research shows that oral medications are frequently not enough for patients to maintain healthy blood sugar. For instance, a 1998 British study of nearly 600 people with type 2 diabetes found that within three years of starting on metformin and a sulfonylurea, just one-third of patients had A1c readings below 7 percent. This is critical, as over the long term, levels higher than 7 percent can lead to organ damage. On the other hand, properly executed insulin therapy is just about foolproof, with a stellar track record for lowering blood sugar.

When blood tests reveal glucose levels that remain stubbornly high, doctors will usually advise insulin therapy. Although many physicians once considered insulin injections to be the treatment of last resort for their patients with type 2 diabetes, many now see this form of hormone replacement therapy as a way to better manage the disease at earlier stages in order to prevent the serious and often debilitating complications that can result from chronically elevated blood sugar.

If your doctor is recommending insulin therapy for you, don't panic. Take a deep, relaxing breath, and turn to the next chapter to read more about this successful approach to reining in out-of-control blood sugar.

# Give Insulin a Shot for Type 2

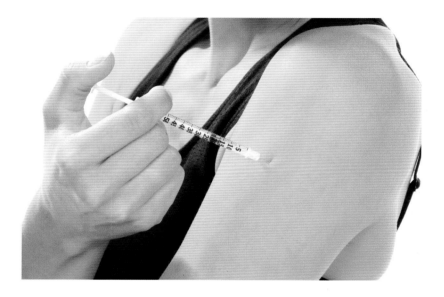

People with type 1 diabetes are well aware of the value of insulin therapy. After all, without the hormone injections, they would die. For folks with type 2 diabetes who have been advised to begin insulin injections, however, fear, misinformation, or uncertainty can keep them from seeing—and taking advantage of—the therapy's very real benefits.

In this chapter we tackle some of the common psychological obstacles that type 2 sufferers can face when considering the addition of insulin therapy to their diabetes treatment plan. And then we explore the practical aspects of choosing and using insulin to improve blood sugar control.

# Overcome Your Fear

When a patient with type 2 diabetes can no longer control blood sugar with diet, exercise, and oral medication, the next obvious step is to begin insulin therapy. However, doctors say that many patients have an emotional response to this news and resist the idea of taking insulin. Indeed, some patients bring a whole new meaning to the phrase "insulin resistance" when their physicians bring up the therapy. They may refuse the treatments because they don't believe they can administer them properly. Or they want nothing to do with needles. Or maybe they associate insulin therapy with their old Aunt Mabel who took the injections but still went blind or ended up in a wheelchair.

When a patient is hesitant or flat-out refuses to take insulin, physicians sometimes say he or she has psychological insulin resistance, or PIR. Several studies reflect the prevalence of PIR. In one large trial, more than one-quarter of type 2 patients who were prescribed insulin refused to take the drug, at least initially. In another, up to three-quarters of patients said they were reluctant to take insulin.

But the longer such therapy is put off, the more damage high blood sugar has a chance to do.

Two experts on diabetes and behavior—William H. Polonsky, Ph.D., of the University of California, San Diego, and Richard A. Jackson, M.D., of Boston's Joslin Diabetes Center—have identified six attitudes and beliefs that can cause PIR. Here they are, followed by a healthy dose of reality:

## 1. Patients view taking insulin as a loss of control.

In one survey, half of patients interviewed said they believed that insulin therapy would restrict or disrupt their lives. Some patients worry that taking insulin will rob their lives of spontaneity, make travel and dining out difficult, and create other hassles. Others worry about the threat of hypoglycemia and weight gain.

**The facts:** The wide variety of insulin available can accommodate most lifestyles and allow for spur-of-the-moment

## You're Not Alone

If your doctor recommends insulin therapy, you're in good company. It's been estimated that between 25 and 40 percent of people with type 2 diabetes inject insulin. Within that group, more than half use only insulin, while the rest take a combination of insulin and one or more other diabetes medications.

changes in plans. Yes, hypoglycemia is a concern, but once a patient learns to manage insulin therapy and oral medications, it is a less common occurrence. Weight gain caused by insulin, if any, is usually modest.

**2.Patients lack confidence in their ability.**
Giving yourself insulin injections is definitely trickier than popping a pill once or twice a day. Not surprisingly, nearly half of patients prescribed insulin worry that they will make mistakes by messing up the timing or delivering the wrong dosage. Unfortunately, self-doubt can turn into a self-fulfilling prophesy, as patients who lack confidence often do a poor of job managing insulin treatments.
**The facts:** Worries about proper technique can be overcome by working closely with your diabetes educator and—as the old saying goes about getting to Carnegie Hall—practice, practice, practice. Using an insulin pen (discussed later in this chapter) instead of a needle may be less intimidating.

**3. Patients feel a sense of failure.**
Patients often say that needing insulin is proof that they did a poor job of taking care of their diabetes. As Polonsky and Jackson explain, "insulin is viewed as a well-deserved punishment for one's own gluttony, sloth, or negligence..."

## Sweet Success

Despite this common aversion to insulin therapy among people with type 2 diabetes, doctors seem to be doing a pretty good job of persuading patients that the treatments are worth the trouble. While the number of type 2-ers who take only insulin has dropped since 1994, the portion using insulin and an oral diabetes drug has tripled and then some.

**The facts:** Diabetes is a chronic disease, and many patients eventually require additional forms of treatment, including insulin therapy. Accepting that possibility early on can eliminate the shock factor if the need arises.

**4. Patients have misconceptions about insulin.**
A patient will often see a prescription for insulin as proof that his or her condition is worsening. Moreover, some patients worry that insulin itself makes you sick. That may be especially true if an older relative lost eyesight or required amputation soon after beginning insulin treatments.

**The facts:** While taking insulin slightly increases the risk of hypoglycemia, there is no truth to myths such as "insulin makes you go blind." When a patient's condition worsens soon after commencing insulin therapy, it's likely that years of poorly controlled blood sugar were the culprit.

**5. Some patients have needle phobia.**
Many patients complain that they don't want—or won't have the guts—to jab themselves with a sharp object several times a day for the rest of their lives.

**The facts:** A mental health counselor can help patients overcome fear of needles. Genuine needle phobia is relatively uncommon. In many cases, patients discover that their anxiety about injecting themselves comes from their frustration with having diabetes.

**6. Patients often have "What's In It for Me?" syndrome.**
A patient who is overcome with doubts and fears about insulin may have a hard time believing the drug's benefits outweigh perceived potential harm. One study found that only one in ten type 2 diabetes patients believed that insulin therapy would improve their health.

**The facts:** Attaining better glucose control through insulin therapy not only reduces the risk for long-term complications, it can also improve mood, energy level, and sleep quality.

# The Ins and Outs of Insulin Therapy

If you are currently taking oral diabetes drugs and your doctor wants you to add insulin to your regimen, you may only have to inject the drug once (probably in the evening or right before going to bed) or twice (morning and evening) a day, at least at first. You and your doctor can select from several different varieties in order to fine-tune your treatment. Some hit your bloodstream and start working right away, while others take their time and last all day. This section provides an overview of the types of insulin available as well as the options for administering it and the importance of rotating injection sites.

# What Kind of Insulin Should You Use?

In the early days of insulin therapy, there was only one variety. After the hormone was injected, it started lowering glucose levels in 60 minutes or less, reached its peak performance within a few hours, then fizzled out, lasting no longer than eight hours. This type, known simply as regular insulin, is still used in diabetes management today.

But scientists eventually figured out that tweaking the amino acids (the building blocks of proteins) in insulin made it

# Insulin: Decisions, Decisions

| TYPE OF INSULIN | EXAMPLES | ONSET OF ACTION | PEAK OF ACTION | DURATION OF ACTION |
|---|---|---|---|---|
| Rapid-acting | Humalog (lispro)<br>NovoLog (aspart)<br>Glulisine (Apidra) | 5 to 15 minutes<br>5 to 15 minutes<br>5 to 15 minutes | 60 minutes<br>30 to 90 minutes<br>30 to 90 minutes | 3 to 5 hours<br>3 to 5 hours<br>3 to 5 hours |
| Short-acting (Regular) | Humulin R<br>Novolin R | 30 to 60 minutes | 2 to 3 hours | 5 to 8 hours |
| Intermediate-acting (NPH) | Humulin N<br>Novolin N<br>Humulin L<br>Novolin L | 1 to 3 hours<br><br>1 to 2.5 hours | 4 to 10 hours<br><br>7 to 15 hours | 10 to 16 hours<br><br>18 to 24 hours |
| Intermediate- and short-acting mixtures | Humulin 50/50<br>Humulin 70/30<br>Humalog Mix 75/25<br>Humalog Mix 50/50<br>Novolin 70/30<br>Novolog Mix 70/30 | Depends on composition of mixture | Depends on composition of mixture | Depends on composition of mixture |
| Long-acting | Ultralente<br>Lantus (glargine)<br>Detemir (Levimir) | 6 to 10 hours<br>2 to 4 hours<br>2 to 4 hours | 10 to 16 hours<br>peakless<br>6 to 14 hours | 18 to 24 hours<br>20 to 24 hours<br>16 to 20 hours |

*All figures are estimates; each user has a unique response to insulin, so the actual time of onset, peak, and duration varies. (The part of the body you use for injection affects times, too.)*

behave differently. In particular, they were able to alter the speed at which insulin is absorbed by the body. The longer it takes your body to absorb a drug, the longer it remains active. This discovery has led to a wider variety of insulin choices that can help you and your doctor tailor your insulin injections to your body's needs.

# Insulin: The Long and Short of It

By tinkering with insulin's molecules, scientists can have been able to alter insulin's speed and durability in three ways:

- Onset: how long it takes the insulin to enter your bloodstream and get to work lowering your blood glucose
- Peak Time: how long it takes insulin to reach maximum strength, when it works hardest
- Duration: how long the insulin works before it quits

The table on page 134 shows the various types of insulin available.

All this variety adds up to several benefits for you. For starters, longer-acting insulin can reduce the number of injections you need in a day. What's more, combining two different types of insulin may help improve glucose control. For example, your doctor might prescribe a long-acting form of insulin called glargine, which has no peak but stays active for 24 hours, slowly letting insulin into your system to maintain daily business. But to accommodate the spike of glucose that hits your system after eating, you may also take a premeal blast of short-acting insulin. Ultimately, the goal is to create a hormonal environment in your body that mimics what your pancreas would do, if only it could.

Premixed insulin represents an option for patients who take two different types of insulin. There are a number of premeasured preparations available that typically blend short- and long-acting forms of insulin or intermediate- and short-acting forms. The goal of using premixed insulin is to reduce the number of injections the patient must make in a day. Premixed insulin has some benefits and downsides, so it isn't for everyone. For example, the convenience of

## The Not-So-Good Old Days

Before modern, disposable needles became available, people with diabetes injected insulin with thick glass needles that had to be sterilized in boiling water every day and sharpened with a pumice stone or razor strap.

## Does Your Doctor Have PIR?

If you believe that insulin therapy is unpleasant and a hassle—even though you don't use it—you may have gotten that impression from your physician. Experts say patients aren't the only ones who can develop psychological insulin resistance. Occasionally, doctors may also be reluctant to put a patient on insulin therapy, whether or not they are conscious of their bias.

There are several reasons a doctor may delay prescribing insulin to patients who need it, according to William H. Polonsky, Ph.D., and Richard A. Jackson, M.D., two leading authorities on PIR. A doctor may:

• anticipate a patient's negative reaction to hearing he or she needs insulin.

• fear the patient will experience frequent bouts of hypoglycemia.

• worry that treating a patient who takes insulin will require more of his or her time.

PIR can be contagious, so your doctor's bias and reluctance may rub off on you. If you have repeatedly failed to meet blood sugar goals, yet your physician has not discussed insulin therapy, ask why.

premixed insulin makes it the best choice for:

• older patients who lack the dexterity to inject themselves or whose memories are too foggy to remember to take insulin on schedule.

• patients who have some trouble with mixing two types of insulin in one syringe.

• patients who find it difficult to make adjustments to their insulin dosages based on changes in their glucose readings.

• patients who still can't find the motivation to inject insulin several times a day despite their doctors' cautions, warnings, and threats

that chronically high blood sugar corrodes arteries and nerves, causing devastating damage to organs and limbs.

Some studies have found that patients (especially senior citizens) make fewer dosing errors when they use premixed insulin instead of mixing two types of insulin on their own. However, while using premixed insulin may seem more convenient, it requires some discipline. For instance, to accommodate the onset, peak, and duration of the two different insulins, the patient must stick to a strict eating schedule and avoid consuming more or less food than planned. Also, some doctors feel that it's very difficult to achieve tight glucose control while using premixed insulin. At best, these blended hormone treatments prevent very high or very low swings in blood sugar.

Advantages of premixed insulin:
- no need to play chemist, since the insulin is mixed for you
- fewer daily injections

Disadvantages of premixed insulin:
- premixed solutions require you to eat a specific amount of food at set times and to strictly adhere to a regular schedule of physical activity
- harder to maintain normal glucose control

# Tools for Injecting Insulin

Wouldn't it be swell if insulin came in an easy-to-swallow pill or maybe a tasty beverage? Unfortunately, tiny, sensitive insulin molecules wouldn't stand a chance in the hostile environs of your stomach, where digestive enzymes would rip them to shreds. That means you have to bypass your gut and deliver this must-have hormone directly into your bloodstream. Traditionally, that has required an injection through the skin.

### Hypodermic Syringes

Just reading those words can make you wince. Your doctor has been jabbing you with these sharp objects since you were a tiny tot. Syringes are cylinders with plungers on one end and hollow needles fitted into the other. Fortunately, the needles used to inject insulin have gone on a crash diet in recent years. They're sharper than ever, too. Slender gauges and finer points mean they hurt less. Some have special slick coatings, too, which let the needle slide under your skin more easily. Anyone who takes insulin will tell you that it's a bigger deal to test your blood glucose than to give yourself a shot. Your doctor or diabetes educator will help you select a syringe that's appropriate for your dose of insulin.

### Insulin "Pens"

Warning: These insulin tools really do look like writing instruments, so don't

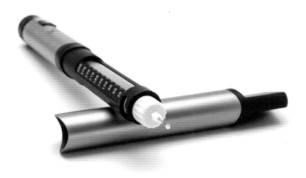

accidentally take out your fountain pen and give yourself a dose of India ink. (The stains will never come out of your arteries.) Like the implements you use for writing, some insulin pens use replaceable cartridges and are designed to be used for a long time; others are disposable (you toss them out after the prefilled pen is empty).

Insulin pens allow you to "dial" the dose of insulin you need. You simply place the tip to your skin and press the plunger to inject. Speaking of tips, here's a good one: When injecting insulin with a pen, count to six slowly before pulling out the needle in order to keep insulin from leaking out of the injection site. (The same advice applies to short syringe needles.) Some people find insulin pens more convenient, especially if they have to inject frequently. What's more, people who use other methods for injecting insulin (such as syringes or pumps) often carry an insulin pen as an emergency backup.

## Jet Injectors

Got a bad case of belonephobia? That's the medical term for fear of needles and other sharp objects. You're in good company; about one person in ten is needle-phobic. An insulin jet injector may be just what you need. These clever tools use high pressure to force a jet stream of insulin through the skin. There is a possible downside, though: Jet injectors can cause bruising.

## Insulin Pumps

Short of an organ transplant (which is an option discussed later in this chapter), an insulin pump is the closest thing to a full-time replacement for a pooped-out pancreas. An insulin pump is a small battery-operated computer, about the size of a pager. (This is a big improvement over the original model introduced in the 1970s, which was strapped onto the patient's back like some sort of George Jetson jet pack.) The computer is attached to a flexible tube with a catheter on the tip. The computer contains an insulin reservoir, and it clips onto a belt, waistband, or some other article of clothing. Using an insertion needle, you place the catheter just under the skin, usually on the abdomen. The process is similar to giving yourself a standard insulin injection, with a big exception: Once you have inserted the catheter, it can remain in place for two or three days before it needs to be replaced and the injection site changed (to prevent infection). And you know what that means—fewer needle jabs.

Based on how much insulin you need and the type you use, you program the computer to deliver an even dose of the hormone (known as basal insulin)

# Rotate Your Injection Sites

If you inject yourself with a needle in the same spot day after day, a funny thing happens: The pierce of the needle hurts less. Even so, you should resist the temptation to establish a permanent pricking point. Here's why: Insulin causes fat to build up. If you inject the same spot with insulin over and over, eventually the surrounding skin can become swollen and lumpy, a condition called lipohypertrophy. It's not just a cosmetic problem, either. Since fat lacks a good supply of blood vessels, it does a poor job of absorbing insulin, so over time your usual dose won't adequately lower your blood sugar. Doctors often find that when long-time diabetes patients who inject insulin develop problems with glucose control, lipohypertrophy is the culprit.

Taking a few simple measures will prevent these unsightly and disruptive lumps. First, rotate your injection sites. There are four spots on your body that are optimal for injecting insulin: Your belly is best—it absorbs insulin fastest. The upper part of your outer arms is the next best choice, followed by your outer thighs. Finally, at the end of the list, is your bottom. These sites make good targets for your needle because they have relatively few nerves and major arteries, which you don't want to puncture.

But don't alternate injection sites willy-nilly. Different types of insulin are absorbed by the body at different speeds, and the site you choose will further influence how fast an injection enters the bloodstream. In general, you may find it best to inject premeal boluses of insulin into the abdomen so they can get right to work, while using your backside for long-acting insulin. Work with your doctor or diabetes educator to create a site-rotation plan.

Here's another rule of thumb: Every time you return to a site, make your injection one inch (or about two finger widths) from the previous injection.

throughout the day. However, for greater flexibility, you can override the computer program with the press of a button and give yourself small doses (called bolus insulin) when necessary, such as immediately before eating. And maybe after eating, too, if you had not planned to have dessert but your willpower crumbled when the waiter uttered the words "chocolate cheesecake." It's easy enough to compensate for the occasional splurge. Some pump manufacturers have even integrated continuous glucose monitoring into their devices, so that users don't have to separately test their blood sugar and

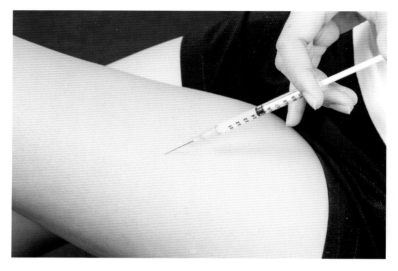

punch in their results multiple times a day. Plus, the more exact control provided by the pump helps prevent hypoglycemia, which can lead to weight gain when extra glucose must be consumed to raise a blood sugar level that's been lowered too far by too much insulin. Studies suggest that people with diabetes who use insulin pumps are better able to manage their blood sugar levels than those who use other methods. That improved management, in turn, can translate into fewer diabetes complications.

Pumps do have a few potential disadvantages, however. Infection is a risk if you don't change the insertion site frequently or get sloppy with your technique. Also, mechanical problems can cause a pump to malfunction, and tubes may become jammed. You could simply run out of insulin and not realize

it. Any one of these problems could cause glucose levels to soar, resulting in a life-threatening condition called ketoacidosis. However, improvements in pump technology make these problems rare.

Insulin pumps are pricey, too—typically in the four figures; however, most health insurers (including Medicare and Medicaid) will cover at least some of the cost.

Perhaps the most obvious problem with insulin pumps is figuring out what to do with the tiny computer when you exercise, sleep, go skinny-dipping, or engage in any other activity where you might find it inconvenient to have an electronic appliance attached to your belly. Most devices, however, can be temporarily disconnected from the injection site so that they won't get in the way or be damaged during such activities.

Despite these potential issues, it's pretty clear that people with diabetes who try the insulin pump find these minor hassles worth tolerating and like the convenience of a device that frees them from making scheduled injections. After all, the insulin pump's popularity rises every year. According to the journal *Postgraduate Medicine*, the number of users in the United States rose from just 6,000 in 1990 to 162,000 by 2001. By 2004, the number of users was estimated at 200,000, and today it's somewhere near 350,000, according to *Diabetes Self-Management*. The magazine further notes that roughly 30,000 of those 350,000 diabetic pump users are thought to have type 2.

## Insulin Inhalers

Pharmaceutical companies have long sought a painfree way to administer insulin, certain that such an invention would be instantly popular among people with diabetes who otherwise have to (or have been advised to) inject the hormone with needles. In mid 2006, the drug maker Pfizer received Food and Drug Administration (FDA) approval to introduce Exubera, the first major alternative to needle injections since the discovery of insulin. Exubera was a form of powdered insulin that patients inhaled through a plastic handheld device similar to the inhalers that are used by people with asthma and allergies. Diabetes patients could use Exubera instead of injecting rapid-acting insulin before meals. Yet the drug didn't catch on, and after less than two years on the market, poor sales forced Pfizer to discontinue the product. Those dismal results also prompted two other drug companies to halt the inhaled-insulin products they had in the works. At least part of the reason that Exubera failed could be traced to the fact that insurers refused to pay for it, saying it was too expensive compared to the standard needle-based delivery systems and that it wasn't effective for a lot of people with diabetes.

Considering the obvious appeal of a needleless insulin delivery system, however, it's not surprising that another company is once again poised to introduce an insulin inhalation system, perhaps as early as 2014. The California-based company MannKind has been working with the FDA since 2009 to gain approval for its inhaled insulin powder, which it calls Afrezza. The inhalation device that will deliver the powder, called Dreamboat, is considerably smaller than the Exubera device: Roughly the size of a child's toy whistle, it fits easily in the palm of the hand. But Afrezza's greatest appeal may be in how quickly and how well it works in people with either type 1 or type 2 diabetes.

# Insulin: A Brief History

Insulin therapy is truly one of the marvels of modern medicine. After all, before the development of injectable insulin, people whose bodies stopped producing the hormone didn't hang around for long. There simply wasn't much doctors could do for them.

In the 19th century, after researchers figured out that the body needs this critical hormone to burn glucose as energy, doctors tried different ways to restart production of insulin in people with type 1 diabetes. Some physicians even tried feeding fresh pancreas to patients. The experiment failed, as did other attempts to replace missing insulin.

Finally, in 1922, a former divinity student named Dr. Frederick Banting figured out how to extract insulin from a dog's pancreas. Banting injected the insulin into the behind of a 14-year-old boy named Leonard Thompson, whose body was so ravaged by diabetes that he weighed only 65 pounds. Little Leonard developed abscesses on his bottom and still felt lousy, but his blood sugar improved slightly. Encouraged, Banting refined the formula for insulin and tried again six weeks later. This time Leonard's condition improved rapidly. His blood sugar dropped from 520 mg/dl to a more manageable 120 mg/dl. He gained weight, and his strength returned.

Banting and a colleague, Dr. John Macleod, won the Nobel Prize for their work. Commercial production of insulin for treating diabetes began soon after. For many years, drug companies derived the hormone using pancreases that came primarily from stockyards, where they were taken from slaughtered cows and pigs.

Despite saving millions of lives over the years, animal insulin has a fault: It causes allergic reactions in some users. To overcome this problem, scientists figured out how to insert the gene for human insulin into bacteria, which in turn churn out pure, high-grade insulin that the human body can't tell from the homemade variety. That's why, since the early 1980s, most people with diabetes who inject insulin have used the human-derived variety.

Recent research indicates that Afrezza is actually more effective than oral diabetes drugs and injectable insulins in matching the way the body's own natural insulin works. When inhaled as the Afrezza powder, the insulin reaches peak levels in 12 to 14 minutes—in other words, in the same amount of time that the body's own insulin peaks in a person who does not have diabetes.

The research further indicates that Afrezza is effective at lowering blood sugar levels in the long term, as measured by A1c testing. And MannKind has said that the cost of its drug could be roughly equivalent to the cost of using one of the insulin pens already that is already on the market.

As with the previous inhaled insulin product, Afrezza may not be appropriate for certain people. If you have asthma or lung disease, for example, or if you smoke, chances are the drug will be off-limits to you. And inhaled formulations in the past were known to sometimes cause a cough or at least a slight loss of lung function.

But if you think you might be interested in this type of insulin delivery system, talk to your doctor about it, and ask him or her to keep you posted on Afrezza's approval status.

# Pancreas and Islet Transplants

As everyone knows by now, when you see a guy in a white coat dashing through a hospital carrying a picnic cooler, he's probably not heading out to a tailgate party at a football game. More likely, he's carrying an organ that has been surgically removed, or "harvested," from a recently deceased donor. Organ transplantation, which once seemed like science fiction, has become common. So why not replace your insulin-poor pancreas with one that's still pumping out plenty of the hormone?

A pancreas transplant can eliminate or reduce the need for daily insulin injections and may prevent (and even reverse) some of the complications that diabetes can cause. But unless you're in pretty bad shape, your doctor probably won't recommend a transplant.

A doctor may recommend a pancreas transplant if a diabetes patient's life is threatened by elevated glucose levels. However, the typical candidate for a new pancreas (new to you, that is) is a person with type 1 diabetes who needs a kidney transplant, too. This situation is hardly unusual, since high, uncontrolled blood sugar can damage the kidneys. Doctors often figure that if they're going to replace a diabetes patient's kidney,

## Two Are Better Than One

The vast majority of pancreas transplants in this country are performed in conjunction with kidney transplants. The organs are usually implanted at the same time (known as simultaneous pancreas-kidney, or SPK). However, in some cases a successful kidney transplant is followed by a pancreas implant (called a pancreas-after-kidney transplant). Research shows that the organs function better when they are both replaced.

Pancreas transplants in the United States:
- 75 percent are simultaneous pancreas-kidney transplants.
- 15 percent are pancreas-after-kidney transplants.
- 10 percent are pancreas-alone transplants.

they may as well throw in a pancreas while they're at it. Having a healthy pancreas may help prevent damage to the implanted kidney. Furthermore, studies show that patients who have a pancreas implanted with a kidney survive longer than patients who only receive a pancreas.

A transplanted pancreas is not a replacement organ, per se, since the surgeon will leave your own pancreas in place; after all, it may not make insulin, but it still produces digestive juices. The transplant is sewn into place in the lower abdomen and attached to blood vessels and the small intestines (or, in some cases, the bladder).

Following surgery, the patient's ever-alert immune system will notice that a foreign object has turned up inside the body, so it will naturally want to attack the new pancreas. To help prevent this internal insurrection from destroying, or "rejecting," a new organ, all transplant patients must take drugs that suppress the immune system for the rest of their lives. As you might imagine, suppressing the immune system can come at a cost. A weakened defense allows infections to flourish, so patients have to be vigilant about fevers, sores, and other unexplained symptoms. Drugs that suppress immunity also increase the risk for some cancers. Organ transplants seem to raise cholesterol levels and blood pressure, too.

Since organ transplants are a major ordeal and carry some serious risks, and since there are effective treatments for diabetes, pancreas-only transplants aren't very common. Surgeons in the United States perform about 120 of the surgeries each year. Combination kidney-pancreas transplants are more common but still account for just over 1,000 surgeries annually. To put the number in perspective, nearly 17,000 kidney transplants were performed in the United States in 2012, according to the National Kidney Foundation.

# Beware Highs and Lows

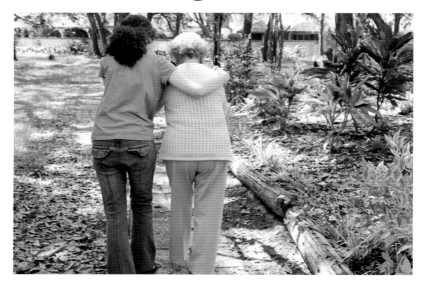

In many aspects of life, success depends on finding the right balance. If you forget the sugar when you bake a birthday cake, for example, it will taste like cardboard. But if you accidentally double the sugar portion, you'll have a treacly torte that's just as inedible. Either way, you won't get many requests for seconds.

Likewise, the key challenge in managing diabetes is keeping your blood sugar in a happy state of equilibrium. Yet, there are many ways to disrupt this balance, including—ironically—taking the very medications you may use to control diabetes. Knowing how to recognize and respond to the symptoms of high and low blood sugar will help keep you blowing out the candles for many years to come.

# Hypoglycemia: The Basics

Keeping blood sugar from rising too high is the goal for anyone with any variety of diabetes. But hypoglycemia is, in a sense, the result of too much success. This term for very low blood sugar is a combination of three Greek words: Hypo = under, glykys = sweet, and haima = blood. Anyone can become hypoglycemic, but for people with diabetes, curbing the threat of nose-diving blood sugar is often just part of daily life.

When glucose levels drop off, cells throughout much of the body can adjust by living off fat and protein, at least temporarily. But one very important organ—the one located between your ears—can't use fat and protein for energy. Since the brain needs glucose to survive, it regards a sugar shortage as a crisis. Early symptoms are no big deal. You feel hungry and a little shaky and nervous, like you had too much coffee. But soon you begin to feel woozy and need to sit down. Your heart thumps, and you break into a cold sweat. Unless you take the proper steps, you may become confused and talk incoherently. Your vision blurs and your head feels ready to burst. In a sense, it is: In extreme cases, hypoglycemia causes convulsions and even comas.

What causes a plunge in blood sugar? In a person who does not have diabetes, hypoglycemia is fairly uncommon, since the body comes equipped with an efficient system that keeps blood sugar levels balanced. When blood sugar begins to drop, the pancreas senses trouble and slows down insulin production, so the body doesn't use up glucose so quickly. For an added boost, the pancreas makes the hormone glucagon, which signals the liver to convert some glycogen (the storage form of sugar, you'll remember) to glucose, then release the sugary stuff into the blood. It all happens so quickly that a dip in blood sugar is brief and goes unnoticed.

But this system can get out of whack if you have diabetes, making it tricky to maintain balanced blood sugar. That's especially true if you inject insulin or take a sulfonylurea or meglitinide, two widely used types of oral medication that perk up insulin production in the pancreas. Getting the proper dose of these therapies exactly right is something of an art. To avoid frequent bouts of hypoglycemia, you must become expert at tweaking your dosage when necessary and knowledgeable about the steps you can take to help keep your blood sugar from plummeting.

# Know the Signs of Low Blood Sugar

Hypoglycemia, or low blood sugar, is a risk for anyone who has diabetes. However, it's most common among patients who inject insulin or take insulin-stimulating drugs, including sulfonylureas and meglitinides. Consider hypoglycemia when you begin to feel any of these symptoms:

- excessive hunger
- nervousness
- the jitters or shakiness
- sweating for no apparent reason
- anxiety
- weakness, loss of coordination
- dizziness or feeling light-headed
- unusual sleepiness
- confusion
- difficulty speaking
- blurred vision

If any of the following occurs while you're in bed, low blood sugar is a possibility:

- You have a nightmare or cry out in your sleep.
- You awaken with your pajamas or bed sheets soaked with perspiration. (Even if there's a chance that your night sweats could be associated with perimenopause, play it safe and check your blood glucose level.)
- In the morning you feel tired, confused, or irritable or you awaken with a headache.

## Preventing Hypoglycemia

Chances are, you are going to experience at least a touch of hypoglycemia now and then. Accepting that these occasional spells are part of coping with diabetes can make them less upsetting or disruptive. Better yet, take the following advice and limit your bouts with low blood sugar.

## Medications

Insulin therapy and insulin-stimulating drugs are lifesavers. But these treatments know how to do one thing—lower blood sugar. Even when glucose levels reach perilously low levels, they keep doing just that, ignoring cues from the body to knock it off.

148

One common cause of hypoglycemia is medication overkill: Even though you took the recommended dose, it was more medicine than your body needed. It's a little bit like extinguishing a lit match with a fire hose.

In other words, you artificially increased insulin levels beyond the amount you needed to control blood sugar. This can occur because you goofed up and took too much medicine, of course. However, often this problem is unavoidable and happens even if you do everything right. Your quirky corpus can change its mind about how much insulin it needs from day to day. You can even monitor your glucose levels with the vigilance of a hawk and still end up having a hypoglycemic episode. (In fact, experts say that people with type 1 diabetes can count on having at least one per week.) Obviously, this can be frustrating and make you wonder whether your efforts are worth it. However, don't give up. Various lifestyle decisions and choices you make every day will affect how well insulin therapies work, as you'll learn when you read on.

One thing you can and should do is discuss with your doctor or diabetes educator how much insulin or insulin-stimulating medication you need and how your lifestyle will affect the dose you should take.

# Meals

Say you are about to head down to the cafeteria for lunch when the boss asks if you faxed that 50-page document to Los Angeles—the one that was supposed to be there an hour ago. Or you're halfway through dinner when your long-lost twin sister Mildred shows up at the door. You are probably not going to say, "Great to see you, Millie, but give me five minutes while I finish this tuna sandwich."

Because you have diabetes, you must be sure that your body has enough insulin to process the food you eat, especially if you inject insulin or take sulfonylureas or meglitinides. But when you skip or put off a meal—or eat less than you planned—you can end up with more insulin than you need.

**Tips:**
- Try to eat meals and snacks at the same time every day.
- Avoid skipping meals.
- Clean your plate—eat as much as you planned. However, if you find that you need to overeat in order to prevent low blood glucose, discuss this with your doctor.
- Talk to your doctor or diabetes educator about what to do on days when interruptions to your meal routine are unavoidable.

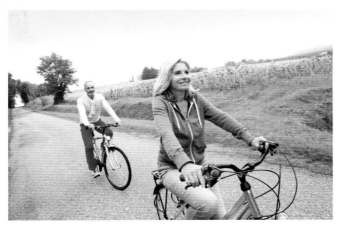

## Exercise and Other Physical Activity

Keeping fit has unquestionable benefits for anyone with diabetes. But if you have diabetes, especially the type 1 variety, exercise requires a bit more planning than simply deciding whether you'll use the stair-climber or elliptical trainer when you get to the gym.

The problem begins with your muscles. During exertion, their fuel demand skyrockets. In a person who does not have diabetes, insulin levels drop and glucagon rises, causing the liver to release glucose so cells can burn it as energy. As a result, blood sugar levels remain fairly constant.

Unfortunately, if you have type 1 diabetes, your pancreas doesn't respond to exercise and the greater demand for glucose by reducing insulin levels because, well, you don't have any insulin to cut back on. Instead, you add insulin to your blood by injecting it. But the dose you need while sitting around the house staring at the fish tank is much higher than what you need while playing full-court basketball. If you don't adjust the dose accordingly, high insulin levels in the blood will prevent your liver from releasing stored glucose and, as a result, your blood sugar levels will fall. Game over.

Exercise-induced hypoglycemia is also a concern for people with type 2 diabetes who take a sulfonylurea or meglitinide. Although your pancreas may want to slow insulin production during exercise, both drugs make sure it continues to pump out the hormone.

In addition, beware another post-workout phenomenon known as delayed hypoglycemia. After exercising, your tired muscles restock themselves with glucose and your liver takes its sweet time rebuilding its inventory of glycogen (the stored form of glucose). While all this is going on, blood sugar can remain low. If you don't eat enough food after strenuous exercise, delayed hypoglycemia can strike—usually between 6 and 15 hours later. But delayed hypoglycemia can

# How to Treat Low Blood Sugar

**If you suspect low blood sugar:**

1. Confirm your hunch by checking your blood sugar. If it's over 70 mg/dl, your blood sugar is okay, but consider what else might be making you feel weird. If your blood sugar is 70 mg/dl or lower, assume you have hypoglycemia. If you can't check your blood sugar but suspect it may be too low, play it safe and take further steps.
2. Eat, drink, or swallow 15 grams of simple sugar.
3. Wait 15 minutes, then check your blood sugar again. If it's above 70 mg/dl, the crisis is averted. If it's still lower than 70 mg/dl, consume another 15 grams of sugar.
4. Wait another 15 minutes, then check your blood sugar. If it's above 70 mg/dl and your next meal is more than 30 minutes (some experts say 60 minutes) away, have a snack that contains carbohydrates, protein, and fat.
5. If your blood sugar doesn't rise above 70 mg/dl, repeat the process until it does. If it remains stubbornly low, call your doctor or go to an emergency room.

Be sure that family, friends, and coworkers can recognize symptoms of hypoglycemia; if you fail to notice and act on them in time, your condition may worsen to the point that you are unable to help yourself. Make sure they know what to do—and what not to do—if you can't swallow, become unconscious, or are unable to treat your hypoglycemia for any reason.

- They should give you a glucagon injection immediately, even if it's not clear you have low blood sugar.
- They should call 911 or the local emergency number if the glucagon doesn't relieve your symptoms.
- They shouldn't attempt to give you insulin or other diabetes medicine.
- They shouldn't attempt to feed you.

actually occur as many as 28 hours after a workout. One study found that over a two-year period, 48 out of approximately 300 young type 1 diabetes patients had a bout with delayed hypoglycemia. The problem may be more likely to occur if you work out more intensely or longer than usual.

**Tips:**

- Talk with your doctor or diabetes educator about adjusting your insulin dose or your snack intake before working out, playing a sport, or participating in any other physical activity that will make you huff and puff.

# The Road to Ruin?

Shaky hands and rattled nerves. Dizziness and blurred vision. Confusion and loss of coordination. A serious episode of hypoglycemia is guaranteed to spoil a leisurely Sunday drive in the country. Although people with diabetes who take the proper precautions can be excellent drivers, studies show that patients who have the disease (especially type 1) can pose a risk on the road.

A 2003 study in *Diabetes Care* found that about one in three people with type 1 diabetes had become hypoglycemic while driving. Not surprisingly, they had more than twice as many accidents as their nondiabetic spouses. The type 1 patients had significantly more traffic violations, too.

Other studies offer clues about how diabetes patients can ensure that when they set off for work in the morning, they don't end up in the emergency room. A 1999 survey in the *Journal of the American Medical Association* found that 45 percent of people with type 1 diabetes said they would be willing to get behind the wheel even if they knew their blood sugar was too low. Another study of 202 motorists with insulin-treated diabetes found that 59 percent said they never test blood sugar before driving.

Whether you have type 1 or type 2, if you are at risk for hypoglycemia, these simple measures can keep you out of accidents and traffic court:

- Always test your blood sugar before driving. If it's too low, don't drive until you have taken the steps outlined in How to Treat Low Blood Sugar on page 151.
- Keep a carbohydrate snack in the car at all times. If you feel the symptoms of hypoglycemia coming on while driving, pull over and attempt to correct your blood sugar.

- Inject insulin in the abdomen before exercise; research shows that flexing, stretching, pumping limb muscles absorb injected insulin too quickly during exercise.
- Plan on having a snack during very long bouts of exercise, such as long-distance running, cross-country skiing, or rowing.
- Monitor, monitor, monitor. Check your blood sugar levels before and after exercising—you can even check during the activity, if you're in the gym or on the track for a long time.
- Consider eating a snack after a long workout to help reduce the risk for delayed hypoglycemia.

## Alcohol

If you know a little about the chemistry of alcoholic beverages, it may seem odd to learn that drinking booze can cause low blood sugar. After all, many forms of alcohol contain carbohydrates, which break down into glucose in the body. A can of beer, for example, contains roughly the same amount of carbs as a piece of taffy. In fact, if you are well fed, drinking a lot of alcohol can have the opposite effect, causing blood sugar to soar too high. (Hyperglycemia is discussed later in this chapter.)

However, drinking alcohol on an empty stomach can cause your blood sugar to plummet. And if you haven't eaten in a while, your blood sugar levels may already be on the low side. Without food to break down into glucose, your liver converts stored glycogen into simple sugar, which it releases into the blood to keep your organs functioning, especially your brain. (Don't forget, your brain cells are fussy eaters that will only consume glucose for energy.)

But tossing back a few glasses of wine when your body is relying on the liver for its supply of glucose can turn happy hour into a horror show. Alcohol interferes with the liver's ability to produce glucose molecules, which can leave the body bereft of its most efficient energy source. Be careful about your alcohol intake—and if you've had problems regulating your blood sugar, opt for a non-alcoholic drink.

**Tips:**

If you want to enjoy an adult beverage or two without sending your blood sugar into a tailspin, follow these rules:

- Check your blood sugar before the first sip. If it's low, either don't have any alcohol or teetotal until you have had something to eat and given your glucose a boost.
- Always drink with a meal or shortly after eating.
- Become a moderate: One drink for women and two for men is the daily max. And the 24-ounce super schooner of ale at your favorite pub counts as two drinks, not one. (A "drink" usually means 12 ounces of beer, 5 ounces of wine, or 1.5 ounces of liquor.) Don't hit the sauce more than one or two days a week.
- Take a break between drinks. If you're at a party and feel funny walking around without a drink, have a tall glass of seltzer with lemon.
- Stick to light beers, dry wine, and cocktails mixed with diet sodas—they contain fewer carbohydrates. Avoid sugary drinks.
- If you become hypoglycemic and start stumbling around or acting confused, your bar mates or fellow partygoers may assume you have had a drink or three too many. Far from wanting to help you, they may try to avoid you. Tell someone in advance that you

have diabetes and may need assistance.

- Alcohol can keep blood sugar suppressed for up to 12 hours, so check your glucose before going to bed. If it's below 100 mg/dl, have a snack.
- Wear a MedicAlert identification or another type of bracelet or necklace that identifies you as someone who has diabetes.

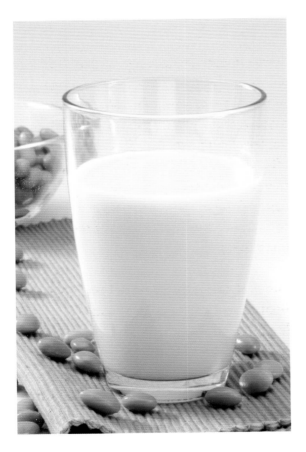

# Sweet Salvation: Treating Hypoglycemia

If you have diabetes and suddenly notice that you feel light-headed and jittery, especially if you use insulin therapy, there's an excellent chance you have developed hypoglycemia. But confirming your suspicion is a good idea, since low blood sugar can occur for other reasons. (See Other Causes of Hypoglycemia, page 156.) Here's yet another good reason to keep your glucose meter handy. If a spot check reveals a glucose reading that's 70 mg/dl or lower, low blood sugar is the culprit.

The solution is surprisingly straightforward. You don't have to take a special drug that triggers your pancreas to produce hormones or that knocks out enzymes responsible for modulating some complex biochemical reaction. Your blood sugar is low, so the goal is to put more into circulation, ASAP. The fastest way to boost glucose is by consuming 15 grams of simple sugars, which break down rapidly in the body. You might have to give yourself another dose if your symptoms don't fade within 15 minutes or so. (See How to Treat Low Blood Sugar on page 151.)

Your medicine chest, nightstand, glove compartment, desk, briefcase, purse, and

Careful planning, with the aid of your doctor or diabetes educator, can help prevent hypoglycemia and make the condition easier to manage when it does arise.

- Know the symptoms of hypoglycemia.
- Try to stick to a regular meal schedule and eat as much food as planned.
- Don't overdo exercise.
- Discuss with your doctor or educator how to adjust insulin or medication doses on occasions when you may eat more or less than planned or may be more active than normal.
- Don't abuse alcohol.
- Have a fast-acting carbohydrate snack, such as a small box of raisins, handy at all times.
- Educate family members, friends, and coworkers about hypoglycemia and what to do if you need their help correcting your blood sugar.
- If you have a glucagon emergency kit, make sure the medicine hasn't expired.

gym bag are all good places to keep a stash of quick fixes for hypoglycemia. Some good choices for boosting low blood sugar include:

- 2 or 3 glucose tablets
- ½ cup of fruit juice
- ½ cup of a regular soft drink (not a diet beverage, which contains no sugar)
- 1 cup of milk
- small boxes of raisins
- 5 or 6 pieces of hard candy
- 1 or 2 teaspoons of honey or sugar
- a tube of glucose gel or other antihypoglycemia product (more about those later)

You might read this list and have a question or two. We'll try to answer!

**Since when is milk a sugar powerhouse?** Surprise! Milk contains a form of simple sugar called lactose. Some people can't digest lactose and end up experiencing unpleasant gastrointestinal problems after consuming it. But if milk doesn't bother you, it can be a healthy source of hypoglycemia-fighting sugars, since it also contains calcium, protein, and other good things.

**Mmm, cheese—that's made from milk, right...?** Nice try, but most cheeses (especially aged varieties, such as cheddar and Swiss) are relatively low in lactose, so they won't raise your blood sugar much.

**Then how about candy bars? They contain a lot of sugar.** They sure do, along

...can hurt you, a lot, if you have diabetes. People who have had the disease for a long time can develop a condition called "hypoglycemia unawareness." As the name suggests, people who have hypoglycemia unawareness have a hard time recognizing familiar symptoms of low blood sugar in themselves. Anyone who takes insulin should have a glucagon emergency kit, but if you feel that you may miss the early clues of hypoglycemia, it's particularly important to keep one handy. Be sure to talk to your doctor about getting a glucagon emergency kit. Glucagon, as you already know, is a hormone that causes the liver to release glucose into the bloodstream. These kits contain a vial of glucagon and a syringe. Be sure to familiarize friends, coworkers, and family members with the symptoms of hypoglycemia, and teach them how to use the syringe in case you experience an episode of severe hypoglycemia and can't help yourself.

with a lot of fat from chocolate, nuts, peanut butter, and other ingredients. Fat slows the absorption of sugar in the gut. Besides, fat is an ultradense source of calories, so restocking your blood with glucose by chowing on chocolate bars will contribute to ultradense hips and thighs.

**Aren't those special hypoglycemia products a rip-off?** Maybe not. Hard candy, raisins, and soft drinks can relieve hypoglycemia effectively. But snack-type foods and beverages can lure you into nonemergency noshing. That is, if your will is weak, you may gobble or gulp them just because you're hungry or thirsty. Not only could you find yourself empty-handed if your blood sugar dips, but the unneeded sugar could cause glucose—along with your weight—to soar. On the other hand, although glucose tablets and gels won't make you gag, you probably won't be tempted to break them out for your midafternoon snack. (The American Diabetes Association Web site at diabetes.org offers a comprehensive list of products for preventing and treating hypoglycemia.)

# Other Causes of Hypoglycemia

Using insulin or insulin-stimulating medications increases the risk for low blood sugar, but the problem can be triggered by other conditions and circumstances. If you develop symptoms but your glucose levels appear to be safe, talk to your doctor. Hypoglycemia can also be caused by:

- other medications, including aspirin, sulfa drugs (for treating infections), pentamidine (for serious pneumonia), and quinine (for malaria)

- alcohol, especially if you go on a bender. Heavy doses of booze interfere with the liver's ability to release glucose.
- other illnesses, including diseases of the heart, kidneys, and liver. Also, rare tumors called insulinomas produce insulin, which would raise levels of the hormone too high, causing blood sugar to drop.
- hormonal deficiencies. More common in children, a shortage of glucagon, as well as other hormones (including cortisol, growth hormone, and epinephrine) can cause hypoglycemia.

Hypoglycemia is rare in children, but it can happen.

## Honk if You Have Hyperglycemia!

Doctors sometimes call this condition hyperosmolar nonketotic coma, even though patients lapse into a coma in fewer than 10 percent of cases. However, this alternative name does allow physicians to refer to the condition by the amusing acronym HONK.

# Hyperglycemia

Astute readers have probably already figured out that if hypoglycemia means too little glucose in the blood, then hyperglycemia must mean too much blood sugar. But isn't that the topic of this entire book? Isn't the basic problem of diabetes that you have too much sugar in your blood?

Yes, but—you guessed it!—the story is a bit more complex. Technically speaking, a doctor could say you have hyperglycemia if a blood test shows that your glucose is higher than it should be (usually defined as more than 100 mg/dl between meals and 140 mg/dl or higher after eating). It's no big deal if your glucose creeps up a little now and then, but chronically elevated blood sugar can be debilitating and potentially fatal. If you don't take the steps discussed in previous chapters for controlling diabetes, you will probably at minimum develop one or more of the complications explained in Chapter 2.

But the term hyperglycemia can also refer to an acute case of very high blood sugar, which you definitely want to avoid, too. Hyperglycemia can lead to two serious conditions. One occurs primarily (though not exclusively) in people with type 1 diabetes, while the other is mostly a concern for type 2 patients.

## Diabetic Ketoacidosis

In Chapter 1, you learned about ketones, which are leftover products your body makes when it burns fat instead of glucose for energy. Any time you shed flab on a weight-loss diet, your body cranks out ketones. You produce a whole lot of ketones on some diets, such as the famous (or infamous, depending on your viewpoint) Atkins plan. Atkins allows only small servings of carbohydrates, dramatically reducing your body's main source of glucose. Still, your cells get some glucose on low-carb diets. In a person who does not have type 1 diabetes—whose pancreas still makes insulin—the concentration of ketones in your body while eating a low-carb diet never poses a serious health threat, other than to drive away friends and loved ones (ketones can

make your breath smell like you brush your teeth with paint thinner).

However, trouble starts if your blood becomes flooded with ketones, which can happen if your body runs very low on insulin. That risk is always a possibility with type 1 diabetes. At first you may simply need to urinate a lot to unload all the glucose you're not burning. Since you're losing so much water in the urine, you'll become thirsty, too. As your blood becomes more saturated with ketones, you will probably begin to feel lousy in all ways—tired, nauseated, feverish. Your heart will race, and you'll pant like a big dog on a hot day. If you don't receive medical attention, you could slip into a coma and die.

Some common causes of diabetic ketoacidosis include:

- Infections. As your body fights bacteria, it produces hormones that interfere with insulin and trigger the liver to release glucose. Urinary tract infections are a common cause of ketoacidosis in patients with type 1 diabetes.
- Stress. Emotions can trigger a similar hormonal onslaught. So can anything that stresses your body, such as trauma, a serious illness, or surgery.
- The "Oops" Factor. As in, "Oops, I forgot to inject insulin before

lunch." (Physicians favor the term "noncompliance.") Some experts say the problem is particularly common among teenagers, though anyone with type 1 diabetes can develop a potentially dangerous case of forgetfulness. Indeed, when ketoacidosis occurs in a patient over and over again, forgetfulness or some other cause of poor compliance is usually to blame.

- Other insulin problems. Patients who use insulin pumps may not notice if the device becomes clogged or for some other reason fails to deliver a scheduled dose, and ketoacidosis could result. Injecting outdated insulin could have the same effect.
- The "I've Got What?" Factor. Did those early symptoms of ketoacidosis—the unslakeable thirst, the well-worn path to the restroom—sound familiar? They should, since they are the early signs of type 1 diabetes. In fact, some patients learn for the first time that they have the disease when they develop ketoacidosis and see a doctor for treatment.

Once again, be glad you weren't born a century ago. Before the discovery of insulin in 1922, ketoacidosis spelled certain doom. Today, ketoacidosis is fatal in fewer than five percent of cases. Treatment focuses not only on restocking your insulin but also on lowering glucose levels, whisking ketones out of the blood, and restoring all the water the condition drains from the body.

And preventing ketoacidosis is as simple as taking a quick trip to the bathroom or doing an additional fingerstick. A urine or blood ketone test can pick up signs of ketoacidosis before the symptoms get out of control. As a rule, it's a good idea to give yourself a ketone test if you meet certain criteria.

## Aim for Balance

The goal for any diabetes patient is tight control of blood sugar. Follow these steps to help prevent glucose levels from dipping or soaring to extremes:

- Know the symptoms of hyperglycemia.
- Monitor your blood sugar regularly. As little as one check per day could spot a case of hyperglycemia before it causes symptoms.
- Ask your doctor or diabetes educator how often and when you should use urine ketone tests.
- If you feel thirsty, drink something—preferably water.

159

- Your blood sugar is higher than 240 mg/dl (some doctors say 300 mg/dl is a better benchmark; ask your physician)
- You become nauseated or start vomiting
- You develop the flu, pneumonia, or any other serious illness
- You are pregnant

Talk to your doctor or diabetes educator about using urine ketone tests to detect ketoacidosis. Specifically, ask how often and when you should check for ketones and what you should do if a test turns up high levels.

# Hyperosmolar Hyperglycemic Syndrome

Despite the name, this condition has nothing to do with your molars. Instead, hyperosmolar hyperglycemic syndrome (HHS for short) occurs for lack of one of the most common elements—the clear, wet stuff that comes out of the tap in your kitchen or in overpriced bottles at the grocery store. Water is a critical player when glucose builds up in the blood. Normally, when blood sugar rises, the kidneys swing into action and lower levels by excreting excess glucose in the urine. But when the body's water supply runs low, the kidneys slow down urine production. Glucose builds up even more, further increasing demand for water.

Some of the symptoms of HHS resemble those of diabetic ketoacidosis, such as increased thirst, fatigue, and weakness. (HHS does not, however, produce paint-thinner breath, since it doesn't cause ketones to flood the blood.) As HHS progresses, patients may develop rapid heartbeat and sunken eyeballs. They may also become confused and move awkwardly. At advanced stages, HHS can lead to convulsions and coma.

In some cases, a glass of water is all it would take to prevent HHS. The condition often strikes elderly patients with type 2 diabetes (HHS is rare in type 1 patients) who become dehydrated because they can't tend to their own thirst or because whoever should be helping them to wet their whistles (nursing home attendants, for example) aren't getting the job done. Some other causes of HHS include:

- poorly treated or undiagnosed type 2 diabetes
- weak kidneys or kidney dialysis
- infections, heart attacks, and strokes—or any other stress on the body, such as surgery
- medications (Certain drugs used to treat hypertension, asthma, and allergies can cause dehydration, block insulin, or raise glucose.)
- vomiting. (Losing your lunch causes dehydration.)

HHS is definitely a medical emergency. Doctors treat the condition with intravenous fluids to rehydrate the body and insulin to bring down soaring glucose levels. However, patients have often lapsed into a coma by the time they arrive in an emergency room. HHS is fatal in up to 40 percent of cases.

As with diabetic acidosis, the key to preventing HHS is vigilant monitoring—in this case with a glucose meter. If levels rise and don't come down, for any reason, contact your physician.

## It Takes All Types

Many doctors believe that diabetic ketoacidosis is rare in patients with type 2 diabetes. There is also a common perception that when the condition does strike a type 2 patient, it's almost always triggered by a stressful event. However, in a 1999 study published in the *Archives of Internal Medicine,* researchers looked up 141 people who had sought treatment for symptoms of hyperglycemia two and a half years after they had been admitted to a hospital in Houston. It turns out that 39 percent of the patients actually had type 2 diabetes. What's more, there was no evidence in half of the cases that stress was the trigger. The moral: If you have any kind of diabetes and develop symptoms of hyperglycemia (such as extreme thirst, a frequent need to urinate, nausea, or vomiting), call your doctor.

# Protect and Prevent

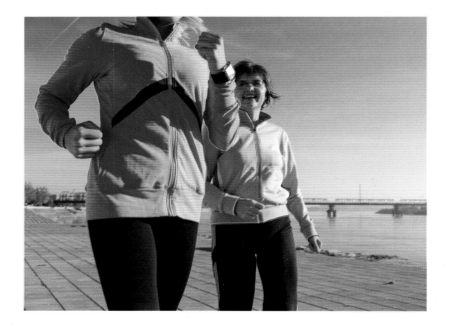

As we have emphasized throughout this book, the ongoing high blood sugar levels of diabetes can cause all sorts of damage throughout your body. That's why it's so important to get them down into a healthy range and keep them there over the long haul. But in addition to your concerted efforts to get your blood sugar under control, there are additional steps you can take to help protect parts of your body that are especially vulnerable to injury and malfunction as a result of your diabetes and to prevent complications.

# Your Eyes and Diabetes

The eyes are the window to the soul, as the old saying goes. Some scientists estimate that when our vision is healthy, we get 70 to 80 percent of our information about the world through our eyes. We hold the gift of vision in such high regard that it has become a metaphor for wisdom and prescience. But when your eyesight goes on the blink (pardon the pun), metaphors aren't much help.

When you were diagnosed with diabetes, one of your first thoughts may have been: Does this mean I'll go blind? It's an understandable fear, since diabetes is the number one cause of blindness. Diabetic retinopathy, the result of damage to the retina caused by high glucose levels, is the leading form of eye disease among people with diabetes, affecting both type 1 and type 2 patients. And its toll has been increasing at an alarming rate. According to Prevent Blindness America and the National Eye Institute, the number of people age 40 and older living with diabetic retinopathy increased 89 percent between 2000 and 2012, to more than 7.5 million Americans. Diabetes increases the risk for other common eye diseases, too. And while aging results in natural changes to the eyes that can diminish vision—which is why reading glasses are a baby boomer fashion staple—diabetes can make matters worse.

# How You See Life

Like so many body parts, the eyes customarily come in matching pairs. (In rare cases, the eyes are not a perfect match; people with a condition called heterochromia have two different-colored irises.) Each eye is roughly one inch in diameter, though only about one-sixth of it is visible; the rest of the orb is tucked into the eye socket. The portion of the eye seen by the outside world resembles a tiny fried egg. The white exterior is connective tissue called the sclera, while the colored center, actually a ring of tiny muscle fibers, is known as the iris. The iris contracts and dilates to alter the size of the pupil, a small, dark opening in the middle of the iris that controls how much light enters the eye.

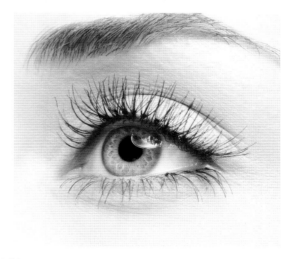

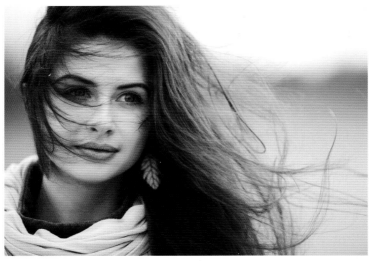

The eye is frequently compared to a camera, with good reason. A thin, transparent shell called the cornea protects the outside of the eye and acts as a lens, focusing incoming light, which is directed to a second lens tucked behind the pupil. This interior lens changes shape to adjust the focus, then bounces light to the back of the eye, where a ring of nerve cells called the retina collects the light, converting it into electrical messages. These messages are then transferred along the optic nerve to the brain, which interprets the world that our eyes see.

## Diabetic Retinopathy

In diabetic retinopathy, damage to the retina from high blood sugar interferes with the eye's ability to send information to the brain. It does not always cause symptoms. Some patients only know they

have diabetic retinopathy because doctors discover evidence of the damage in an eye exam. However, the condition can lead to severe vision loss. In one study, 3.6 percent of patients with type 1 diabetes were legally blind, while about half as many type 2 patients had the same degree of vision loss. The National Eye Institute classifies four stages of diabetic retinopathy:

**Mild nonproliferative retinopathy.** The blood vessels in the retina may begin to swell and develop small bulges. Doctors call these bulges microaneurysms, because they resemble the blood vessel abnormalities that cause brain aneurysms. Blood vessels may leak blood or fluid, forming deposits called exudates.

**Moderate nonproliferative retinopathy.** Diabetes causes blockages in blood vessels throughout the body, and those within the eye are no exception. As retinopathy worsens, the tiny blood vessels that nourish the retina start to clog.

**Severe nonproliferative retinopathy.** At this stage, so many blood vessels in the retina become blocked that parts of the retina begin to starve. In a panic, the eye signals the brain to build new blood vessels to renourish the deprived parts.

**Proliferative retinopathy.** The brain triggers the growth of new blood vessels, a process called neovascularization. But the new vessels are weak and abnormal. Nonproliferative retinopathy (sometimes called background retinopathy) may be very mild. A patient may not notice any vision changes and only learn of a problem during an eye exam. However, as blood vessels begin to leak into the retina, vision may blur. Problems become more serious if leaky blood vessels cause the macula, an area of the retina, to swell, interfering with the ability to see fine details. When severe, this problem, called macular edema, can cause blindness. Vision may blur further as the capillaries, or small blood vessels, feeding the macula become blocked.

Proliferative retinopathy gets its name from the way new blood vessels proliferate, or grow rapidly, in the eyes to compensate for blocked or damaged blood vessels. Unfortunately, these frail replacement vessels do far more harm than good. They do a poor job of supplying blood, and these new vessels can break down and leak (or hemorrhage) into the vitreous, a gel-like substance in the center of the eye. A minor leak may result only in the appearance of a few "floaters" (spots that dance before your eyes). A major vitreous hemorrhage can cause significant vision loss and even blindness. The growth of new blood vessels can also produce scarring that may cause the retina to wrinkle or become detached, further damaging eyesight.

# Other Eye Problems

Two other eye diseases that hit the diabetic population especially hard are glaucoma and cataracts.

**Glaucoma.** This disease, which is estimated to afflict between two and three million Americans age 40 and older, is a leading cause of blindness in the United States. Glaucoma occurs when fluid fails to drain properly from the eyes, causing pressure to build and damage the optic nerve. There are several types of glaucoma. Diabetes raises the risk for neovascular glaucoma, a rare form of the disease. Diabetic retinopathy may cause the growth of new blood vessels on the iris, shutting off the flow of fluid and increasing pressure inside the eye. People with diabetes may be up to twice as likely to develop glaucoma as the general public.

**Cataracts.** More than 24 million Americans age 40 and older have

# Optometrist or Ophthalmologist: What's the Difference?

There are two types of eye care professionals who are qualified to examine your peepers for problems. Understanding the differences in their education and training can help you decide which professional to see.

An optometrist, or doctor of optometry, has an O.D. after his or her name. If you wear eyeglasses or contact lenses, you probably had your eyes examined by—and received the prescription for your lenses from—an optometrist. (However, you probably purchased your glasses from an optician; in some states, opticians dispense contact lenses, too.) Optometrists are not medical doctors but must have an undergraduate degree and then complete a four-year program at an accredited optometry school. Although they do not perform surgery, optometrists can treat patients before and after eye operations. They can also prescribe medications for your eyes.

An ophthalmologist, on the other hand, is a medical doctor (M.D.) or doctor of osteopathy (D.O., who receives similar education as a medical doctor, with additional training in "manual medicine," or manipulation of the muscles and bones). In addition to a bachelor's degree, an ophthalmologist attends four years of medical school, followed by a one-year internship and three-year residency. Ophthalmologists can conduct eye exams, treat diseases and injuries, perform surgery, and prescribe drugs.

You can receive excellent care and treatment from either an optometrist or ophthalmologist. Your physician or diabetes educator may be able to help you locate an eye doctor who specializes in working with diabetes patients.

cataracts, and half of Americans older than 80 have one or have had cataract surgery. Yet diabetes patients are still 60 percent more likely than others to develop this eye disorder. A cataract is a cloudiness caused by changes to fibers in the eye lens. Although a cataract may not cause complete blindness, it can block enough light to obscure visual details and clarity.

## Seeing to Your Eyes

Maintaining tight control of your blood sugar can go a long way toward protecting your eyes. A study called the Diabetes Control and Complications

Trial showed that aggressive insulin therapy dramatically reduces the risk of vision loss. In that study, researchers compared type 1 diabetes patients who gave themselves three or more insulin injections per day (or had an insulin pump) to another group of patients who received one or two insulin injections daily. At the start of the study, none of the patients had signs of retinopathy. After an average of 6.5 years, patients in the aggressive-treatment group were 76 percent less likely to have developed retinopathy. (In an accompanying trial, patients who started with mild signs of retina damage cut in half their risk of further vision loss if they received aggressive insulin treatment.)

In addition, the following steps can help you preserve your sight.

**Be on the lookout for trouble.** Early signs that you may be developing diabetic retinopathy or another issues with your eyes include:
- blurry or hazy vision
- "floaters" or spots that dance before your eyes
- night blindness
- increased sensitivity to glare, especially at night
- double vision
- loss of peripheral (side) vision

- difficulty reading
- a feeling of pressure in the eyes

If you notice any of these signs or any other changes in your vision, see your eye care professional as soon as possible. Don't dismiss vision problems as the effects of fatigue or aging, especially if they are persistent or seem to be getting worse. Early detection and intervention can often keep problems from worsening and preserve your remaining eyesight.

**Have regular eye exams.** Damage to the eye's blood supply that leads to vision loss can go on for years before symptoms arise, so regular examinations are critical. The American Diabetes Association recommends that all patients with type 1 disease undergo comprehensive screening for retinopathy within five years of being diagnosed with diabetes. Type 2 patients should have their eyes thoroughly examined soon after they are diagnosed with diabetes. All diabetes patients should have an annual eye exam unless advised otherwise by their eye care professional. Eye exams should be performed by an optometrist or ophthalmologist. (See Optometrist or Ophthalmologist: What's the Difference? on page 166.) If possible, find one who has experience in diagnosing and treating people with diabetes.

**Lower your blood pressure.** There are plenty of good reasons to keep blood pressure under control, such as lowering the risk for heart disease and stroke. However, high blood pressure also damages blood vessels in the retina, setting the stage for retinopathy. A large British study of more than 1,100 type 2 diabetes patients found that lowering high blood pressure reduced the risk of retinopathy by 34 percent over an eight-year period. Patients who maintained healthy blood pressure had sharper vision, too. (Not surprisingly, they also had fewer heart attacks and strokes.) So if you suffer from high blood pressure, be diligent about following your doctor's orders for treating it, including altering your diet, exercising regularly, and taking medications as prescribed.

**Don't smoke.** And not just because all those clouds of smoke produced by puffing can obscure your vision. Tobacco users have a higher risk of diabetic retinopathy (and a seemingly endless list of other medical problems). If you have diabetes and care about your health (not to mention the well-being of those around you), you've got no business smoking or using any other form of tobacco.

## Practice Your Foot Work

Avoiding foot ulcers and other diabetes complications that affect the lower limbs means following general, big-picture health advice (such as watching your weight and eschewing tobacco) and paying attention to the little details, such as keeping an eye out for tiny cuts and bumps that might turn into large, limb-threatening wounds. These rules can help:

- Keep your blood glucose under control.
- Have your physician check your feet often; undergo a comprehensive examination at least once a year.
- Give yourself a daily foot exam; learn what signs to look for and report anything suspicious to your doctor.
- Maintain a healthy weight and low cholesterol.
- Don't smoke.
- Exercise regularly to help preserve good blood circulation; develop a suitable regimen with your physician.
- Learn the proper way to trim your toenails—or have your podiatrist trim them for you.
- Wear comfortable shoes (and socks or hose) that fit and protect your feet. Don't go barefoot.

## Your Feet and Diabetes

Your feet are surprisingly complex structures. The two combined hold more than one-quarter of the bones in your body—26 each. And while they serve as a solid foundation, the feet aren't static blocks. Rather, they're agile and dynamic machines of movement, with more than 100 tendons, muscles, and ligaments apiece. Given all those moving parts and the pounding that the feet take every day, it's not surprising that, according to the American Podiatric Medical Association, about 75 percent of Americans experience one foot condition or another in their lifetime.

Add diabetes to the mix, however, and the pressure on the feet can become unbearable. Having the condition doubles a person's risk for foot disease. In fact, about 30 percent of people with diabetes who are older than 40 develop medical problems with their feet. And while blood sugar problems can create a dizzying range of hard-to-treat complications throughout the body, those that affect the lower legs and feet can progress with what seems like lightning speed. Indeed, in people with diabetes, lower-limb diseases that are not properly treated can deteriorate so quickly and so badly that doctors have no other choice but to remove the affected area in order to save their patients' lives. The sad result: People with diabetes account for more than 60 percent of all

## Who Gets Foot Ulcers?

Having diabetes increases the chances of developing serious sores on the feet. But some patients have a greater risk than others. To find out what qualities increase the risk, doctors at the University of Washington studied 749 veterans with diabetes. At the outset, none of the veterans had foot ulcers. After an average of 3.7 years, the doctors reexamined the veterans and their medical records. Patients with the following traits were among the most likely to have developed foot sores:

- evidence of nerve damage
- insulin use
- foot deformities, such as hammertoe
- poor vision
- obesity

lower-limb amputations in the United States. A person with diabetes is 10 to 30 times more likely to have a lower limb amputated than is a person who does not have the disease.

As you know all too well by now, the chronically elevated glucose levels of diabetes can damage the nervous system, the wiring that transmits signals from the brain throughout the body. The nervous system works the other way, too: It detects information about the environment and how it affects the body through the five senses. Damaged nerves, or neuropathy, can lead to an array of physical problems and disabilities anywhere in the body. But nerve injuries and other diseases that affect the feet and lower legs may be the complications most frequently associated with diabetes. What's more, the various foot conditions linked to diabetes may be the complications patients dread most.

Annoying and painful symptoms can occur when the brain can't successfully send messages to the feet. But the even greater threat posed by diabetic neuropathy happens when the feet can't send information to the brain because they've become numb from overexposure to blood sugar. Blisters, cuts, and other injuries that once would have made you wince or howl in pain go unnoticed when your feet lose their feeling.

To make matters worse, dulled nerves probably aren't your only problem if you have diabetes. The disease can also cause poor blood circulation. Like the heart's arteries, blood vessels elsewhere in the body can become stiff and narrowed. In fact, 1 in 3 diabetes sufferers over the age of 50 has clogged arteries in the legs, a condition known as peripheral artery disease or peripheral vascular disease. Narrowed arteries diminish blood flow to the lower legs and feet, which can cause pain during long-distance walks. More ominously, the loss of blood flow to the feet can prevent wounds and sores from getting the oxygen and nutrients required for healing, allowing these injuries to fester and spread.

So while occasional bumps, blisters, or cuts on the feet are trivial medical concerns for most people, for diabetes patients these minor injuries can turn serious in a hurry. Left unnoticed and untreated, minor sores on the skin of the foot can turn into severe problems with potentially devastating consequences—namely, foot ulcers.

# Foot Ulcers

Most people think of ulcers as burning sores that cause bellyaches. But while gastric and peptic ulcers that form in the stomach and intestines are usually easy to cure with drugs, ulcers on the skin of the feet and legs can pose a more serious threat. These craterlike wounds can arise from seemingly inconsequential injuries to the feet. In extreme cases, they can deteriorate and develop into crippling complications.

According to the Centers for Disease Control and Prevention, about 15 percent of people with diabetes develop foot ulcers. The problems begin with nerve damage. Specifically, ulcers arise due to a loss of sensation in the foot caused by peripheral neuropathy. (About 60 to 70 percent of people with diabetes have some form of neuropathy.) If feeling in the lower limbs is lost, the risk of foot ulcers soars 700 percent.

When you lose sensation in the feet, small injuries can go unnoticed and degenerate into large, open sores. There are endless scenarios for how a foot ulcer may begin to form, including the following:

- If you have damaged nerves in the lower limbs, you may not be aware that a pair of ill-fitting shoes is causing blisters, corns, or other foot conditions that can lead to ulcers.
- If your skin can no longer distinguish hot from cold, you could scald your foot in steaming-hot bathwater; the burned skin may then blister.
- You could step on a sharp rock or bit of glass and cut your heel while walking barefoot.
- If your foot is numb from nerve damage, you may frequently bang it into hard objects without knowing it because you don't feel any pain. Over time, damage to joints and other structures in the foot could cause a deformity that puts pressure on the skin.
- If you have arthritis in the ankle or toes, you may lose joint mobility and

alter the way you walk so that too much pressure is placed on the ball of the foot. Or, your normal gait may simply apply excessive force on certain sections of your soles. Over time, wear and tear could cause the skin to erode, forming a sore.

- Simply cutting your toenails the wrong way can damage skin and produce sores.

In addition to nerve damage, people with diabetes tend to have several other problems that further increase the risk of foot ulcers, such as:

- Poor blood flow. As mentioned, peripheral artery disease may reduce or cut off blood flow to the lower limbs, which will slow or prevent healing of sores (as well as make walking around the block a painful experience).
- Sugar-rich blood. Bacteria feast on glucose, so the combination of an open wound and high blood sugar can lead to raging infection.
- Decreased immune function. To make matters worse, diabetes interferes with the immune system's ability to kill germs, and that allows infections to worsen.
- Poor vision. If blood sugar has damaged your optic nerves, blurry vision can make detecting cuts and sores more difficult.

## What Is a Podiatrist?

Podiatrists (sometimes known as "chiropodists") are specialized doctors who treat disorders of the foot, ankle, and lower leg, including the various diseases and injuries that frequently afflict people with diabetes. Instead of an M.D., for "medical doctor," they add a D.P.M. after their names, for "doctor of podiatric medicine." But first they must complete four years of extensive medical education and training, including courses in anatomy, chemistry, pathology, and pharmacology. Podiatry students also perform clinical rotations in private practices, hospitals, and clinics. Most states require podiatrists to complete a one- to three-year postdoctoral residency program, too. Finally, before a podiatrist can hang a shingle, he or she must pass an oral and written licensing exam.

- Excess body fat. If you're overweight, as many type 2 diabetes patients are, simply bending over to examine or treat your feet may be difficult, if not impossible.

Foot ulcers and the complications they can cause are not an inevitable part of having diabetes, however. Along with maintaining healthy blood sugar, you can take some additional steps to keep these nasty sores at bay.

**Meet your feet.** Get to know them intimately. Make a point of examining your feet at least once a day. Be on the lookout for any cracks, cuts, sores, bumps, or bruises. Be sure to check between your toes. If necessary, use a hand mirror with a long handle or place a mirror on the floor to check areas that are hard to see. Report any problems to your doctor. If you have poor vision, ask someone else to give your feet a once-over.

**Clean up your act.** Washing your feet daily will do more than keep them from smelling like, well, feet. Good foot hygiene can help prevent infections. To avoid burns, be sure to test water temperature with your hand before stepping into a bath or—better yet—use a thermometer; 90 to 95 degrees Fahrenheit should be about right. Use mild, nonabrasive, unscented soap that contains lanolin, a moisturizer. Dry each foot carefully with a clean towel, especially between the toes. Most doctors discourage patients with foot ulcers from soaking their feet for too long because it robs the skin of its natural protective oils and, ironically, can actually result in dry skin.

**Wear sensible shoes.** "These shoes are killing me!" is the familiar refrain from sore-footed sorts after a day of wearing too-tight pumps or wingtips. While uncomfortable shoes may not be deadly weapons, they can cause foot problems that may turn serious if left untreated. One study of 669 patients with foot ulcers found that about 20 percent of the sores were linked to ill-fitting footwear that caused rubbing on the skin.

A good pair of shoes should be snug but comfortable, without pinching, producing friction against the foot, or cramming the toes together. To find shoes that fit well:

- Shop for new shoes in the afternoon or evening, since your feet swell slightly during the day.

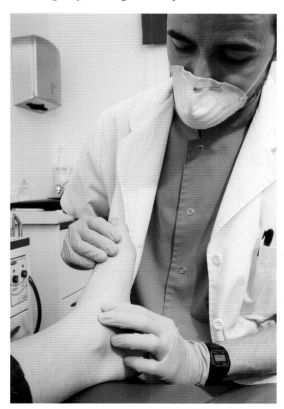

- When shopping for new shows, wear the socks or hose you intend to wear with them.
- Have both feet measured every time you need to buy new shoes. The size and shape of your feet can change over time, and your two feet may not actually be the same size. If your feet are different sizes, buy a pair of shoes that fits the longer and/or wider foot.
- Be sure to try on both the right and left shoe. You want a half inch of space—but not much more—between the end of your longest toe (which may or may not be your big toe) and the front of the shoe. Walk around the store (preferably on both carpet and hard floor) while wearing the shoes to ensure proper fit and comfort before you buy.
- Although you don't have to stomp around in work boots, be sure to choose styles that protect your sensitive feet.
- Avoid sandals and shoes with a thonglike strap between the toes.
- Don't buy an uncomfortable pair of shoes—no matter how much you love the way they look or how "in" they are—in the hopes that they will feel better once you "break them in." Properly fitting shoes should feel good from the get-go.

Therapeutic shoes and inserts may help prevent pressure sores from developing. Specially designed shoes do not eliminate the risk of ulcers, however, and some studies suggest that they may be most beneficial to patients with severe lower-limb problems, such as foot deformities, or to those who have already had a foot amputated. Before purchasing any type of therapeutic footwear, ask your podiatrist whether they are likely to be beneficial for you and what features to look for.

## Cutting Edge Nail Care

Understanding the proper way to care for your nails can spare your feet a lot of grief. Cutting them improperly can promote ingrown toenails, which can lead to infections and ulcers. In fact, some doctors discourage patients with diabetes from using toenail scissors or trimmers at all. One slip and you could cut your skin, opening the door to infection. If you do trim your toenails, follow these rules:

- Cut across the top in a straight line, no shorter than the front edge of the toe.
- Use an emery board to file down sharp corners.
- Never trim the sides of a nail; it exposes sensitive skin to puncturing by the nail.

**Get hosed.** Wearing stockings or socks will help prevent foot problems. When selecting hosiery:

- Opt for those that help your feet stay dry. There is considerable disagreement over whether natural fibers, such as cotton and wool, or specially made synthetic fibers designed to wick moisture away will keep feet driest; your best bet may be to experiment and see which works best for your feet.
- Stay away from tight socks or hose, which can reduce circulation.
- Check that any seams are not bunched up between your toes and inside of the shoe, which can cause blisters.
- No matter what type of socks or hose you wear, change them once a day (or more often if your feet sweat a lot).

**Don't go barefoot in the park.** Or in the backyard, or on the beach, or anywhere else, for that matter, including inside your own home. Hot pavement or sand can burn your feet, sharp pebbles or shards of glass can cause gashes, and you can accidentally stub your toe or kick a hard object just about anywhere. When you're at the beach, lake, or ocean, wear beach or water shoes, which offer more protection than flip-flops. (Wear them at public locker rooms and pools, too, to protect against viruses and fungi.) Find a sturdy pair of slippers to wear around the house.

**Get 'em checked regularly.** Plan on having a thorough foot exam at least once a year, more often if you smoke or have any other condition that raises the risk of ulcers and complications. If you have been diagnosed with neuropathy, ask your physician to have a look at your feet every chance you get. As a reminder for both you and your doctor, take your shoes and socks off as soon as you're shown to the exam table.

# Other Common Foot Problems

Diabetes patients have an unusually high number of foot problems, including those described below. Many of these nuisances can deteriorate into sores that may cause serious foot ulcers. Fortunately, following the daily care suggestions detailed for foot ulcers can reduce the risk for these nagging foot woes, too.

**Athlete's foot.** A notorious menace in locker rooms, athlete's foot is a risk for anyone who does a lot of sweating. Moisture between the toes promotes the growth and spread of fungus. The skin between the digits can become dry, scaly, itchy, and sore. The skin may crack, opening the door to bacterial infection. Blisters may form, too. Over-the-counter antifungal creams are usually effective in treating the condition. But if you don't see improvement in five days or so, contact your doctor.

**Blisters.** These familiar sores form when skin rubs against another surface for an extended period. Over time, layers of skin beneath the area that's rubbing become damaged and blood vessels leak fluid called serum, which collects just under the top layer of skin. (Other influences, such as sunburn and certain diseases, can cause blisters to form, too.) Never pop a blister. Instead, cover it with a sterile gauze pad and bandage. Leave it alone, and the body will eventually reabsorb the fluid. The blistered skin will slide off on its own, probably while you're bathing. If a blister opens, wash it with soap and water, then cover it with gauze and a bandage.

**Charcot's joint.** If nerve damage in the foot is severe enough, you may be able to bang it against the wall or a table leg and not feel a thing. Unfortunately, being impervious to pain may mask mounting damage to joints in the foot caused by a series of minor injuries. Over time, a joint may become so damaged that it stiffens and becomes deformed. Named for a nineteenth-century French neurologist, this condition can affect any joint, though it occurs most frequently in the foot (which is called Charcot's foot). About 15 percent of people with diabetes develop Charcot's joint, which is also known as neuropathic joint or neuropathic arthropathy. A surgeon can remove abnormal bone growth and fragments of cartilage in a procedure known as an ostectomy. The surgeon may also insert screws and plates to realign and stabilize a weakened joint.

**Corns.** If you swear your feet are size 6s when they're really size 7s, you may develop corns as proof of your denial. When you cram your feet into tight shoes, the toes may end up jammed against the inside. As protection against all that pressure and friction, the skin thickens with dead skin cells, which may eventually form small, pea-shape bumps on the tops and sides of the toes. (So why not call them "peas"? Because the layer of skin that accumulates to form a corn is called the stratum *corneum*.) People who have high arches are more at risk for corns, since the shape of their feet adds pressure on the toes. Some corns are painless, while others hurt like heck. Soft toe pads or cushions, available in pharmacies, may help relieve pressure that causes a corn to hurt. Moleskin works, too. But avoid corn remover treatments, which contain acid and may damage your skin. And don't even think about playing amateur surgeon. If a corn needs to be trimmed, let a doctor do the cutting.

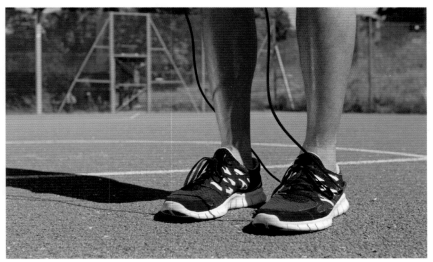

doesn't realize it needs to retain enough water to keep the tissue hydrated. When skin becomes very dry, it may crack, creating an open door for bacteria and other germs and raising the risk of infection. To treat dry skin on the feet, apply a small amount of moisturizing cream or lotion once or twice a day, but avoid the spaces between the toes.

**Calluses.** Like corns, calluses are areas of thickened skin created by friction. They can turn up anywhere on the body, but they usually form over joints and other bony parts. On the feet, calluses most often appear on the soles, often in joggers, walkers, and other people who pound a lot of pavement. Some calluses are painless, while others hurt and may mask the presence of a foot ulcer. Special pads and shoe inserts may help relieve pain, if any. Some doctors recommend smoothing the callus with a pumice stone, but others say the risk of injury is too great, especially if you have diabetes. As with corns, do not attempt to remove a callus with a knife or blade. That's why your doctor gets the big bucks.

**Dry skin.** Damage to nerves in the feet can block signals to the brain. That means the skin may lose moisture, since the body

**Ingrown toenails.** Ingrown toenails may sound like no big deal, but if they aren't treated promptly and properly, they can be a nightmare for people with diabetes. They can occur if the nail becomes deformed and its edge grows inward, pushing its way into the skin. In other cases, the skin on the big toe grows too much and overwhelms the nail. Wearing too-tight shoes is a common cause of ingrown toenails. Improper nail trimming is a problem, too. While a strange-shaped toenail alone is of little consequence and probably won't cause symptoms, an ingrown toenail can become painful and inflamed if the skin becomes infected. To prevent and treat ingrown toenails, wear comfortable shoes that don't strangle your feet. Learn proper nail-trimming technique from your doctor or diabetes educator. (See "Cutting Edge Nail Care" on page 174.) And if a toenail is digging into your skin, don't attempt at-home surgery; ask your doctor to trim it. Should infection be present, you'll be given a prescription for an antibiotic.

**Bunions.** Once again, tight shoes, especially narrow high heels, are the most common cause of bunions; not surprisingly, 90 percent of bunion sufferers are women. In fact, according to the American Academy of Orthopaedic Surgeons, about half the women in the United States have a bunion. (But the problem seems to run in families, too.) Bunions occur when the metatarsophalangeal joint—the joint at the base of your big toe—rubs against the side of your shoe, becomes swollen, and begins to jut outward. That forces the big toe to push inward on the second toe. A domino effect may happen, in which the second toe leans in on the third toe. The swollen joint is usually quite painful, especially when you walk, and can become infected. (A bunionette is a small swollen lump on the outside of your foot, below the little toe. Like its big brother, a bunionette can usually be traced to tight shoes.) The first step your doctor orders to treat a bunion may be

to clean out your shoe closet, or at least get rid of any footwear with pointy toes or heels over 21/4 inches. In severe cases, surgery can realign the bones, tendons, and other structures inside the foot that have shifted out of position.

**Hammertoe.** Although it sounds like what you get if you drop a heavy tool on your foot, hammertoe is yet another deformity that can result from ill-fitting or tight shoes, especially if they squish the toes. Muscle abnormalities in the toes can cause the problem, too. When the front of the foot has to fit into a narrow space, the second, third, and fourth toes may be forced to arch upward to make room. Over time, the muscles in the toe freeze, leaving the digit in a hook, or clawlike, position. The toe may also ache and develop a corn. If you develop hammertoe, your doctor may instruct you to do exercises to strengthen the toe muscles, such as using your foot digits to pick up small objects. Corn pads may help relieve some discomfort. If switching to roomier shoes doesn't solve the problem, minor surgery may be necessary to repair the problem.

**Plantar warts.** All warts are caused by a virus, known as human papillomavirus, that can lurk on floors where people tend to walk around barefoot. But that's where the similarity ends between plantar

If you have always wanted to splurge on a full-length mirror, now would be the time. A good handheld mirror would help, too. Using these tools to examine every inch of your skin daily can help detect small problems before they turn really ugly. Talk to your doctor if any of the following skin changes occurs and persists:

- itchiness
- redness, inflammation
- scaliness
- lumps, especially if they leak discharge (which is a nicer word than "pus")
- pain
- discoloration, blotches, or any other changes in appearance
- blisters
- shininess, hair loss
- thickened areas

warts and warts that turn up elsewhere on the body. Plantar refers to the sole of the foot, where these warts grow. While other warts are round growths that protrude from the skin, plantar warts are flat, since you spend all day standing on them. And while warts elsewhere on the body are painless (if a bit unsightly), plantar warts may hurt, especially when you walk. They may also become infected or bleed. Plantar warts often go away on their own, but if you have one that's painful or persistent, do not attempt to remove it yourself. Do not perform bathroom surgery, and do not use over-the-counter wart treatments, because they can contain harsh chemicals. If your blood glucose control is poor, you can get into trouble rapidly. See a doctor for any foot problems. Your doctor may apply a mild acid solution that can shrink warts or remove the growth with a scalpel or by freezing it (a technique known as cryotherapy).

## Your Skin and Diabetes

If you are tempted to flip past this chapter because you think skin care is for sissies, think again, buster. Skin damage is a major complication of diabetes, with the potential to produce everything from barely noticeable blemishes to disfiguring scars. What's more, maintaining healthy skin is crucial for warding off disease and protecting your innards from the perils of the outside world.

As a matter of fact, every diabetes patient should get to know his or her skin better. By examining yourself every day, from head to toe, you may be able to spot small problems before they turn into serious ones. And, as you'll learn, the skin problems described in the

## Is It Your Meds?

Many commonly prescribed drugs can cause dry skin. Talk to your physician if your skin is parched and you take prescription medications, especially any of these:

- Statin drugs, such as atorvastatin (Lipitor) and simvastatin (Zocor), which lower cholesterol
- Nicotinic acid (niacin), used to increase HDL ("good") cholesterol
- Diuretics, used to lower blood pressure
- Isotretinoin, prescribed to treat acne
- Etretinate (Tegison), prescribed to treat psoriasis.

following pages can serve as a caution that greater health concerns may lie beneath the surface.

Diabetes patients do not have a monopoly on skin problems, of course. Walk into any pharmacy or supermarket and you will find aisles overflowing with emollients, creams, astringents, and salves—evidence that damaged skin is a consuming cosmetic and medical concern for the general population. However, diabetes appears to increase the risk for rashes, sores, and other skin conditions.

According to the American Diabetes Association, about one-third of patients will develop a skin disorder at some point. And as you just learned, the skin on your lower extremities is particularly vulnerable to problems.

## The Skin You're In

As every child learns in school, the skin is the largest organ in the body. Your hide has a surface area of about two square yards and weighs about 10 pounds. Technically, you could say that the skin is the largest organ on the body, since it acts as a protective covering for your bones, muscles, and organs. However, the skin is more than mere armor, with many of its critical roles performed below the exterior.

The body's outer shell, called the epidermis, is made up of a top layer of skin cells that are dead. That's just as well, since they are constantly flaking and peeling off anyway. Fortunately, the body replaces these so-called horny cells just as quickly with new ones, as cells in the lower layer of the epidermis divide. Some cells in the epidermis produce melanin, the pigment that provides skin color. Beneath the epidermis lies the dermis. Hidden from sight, this layer is packed with vital equipment that keeps the skin healthy and performs various functions. In the health-and-beauty department, there are hair follicles and sebaceous glands, which produce oil called sebum that moistens the skin. The dermis also contains nerve endings, which detect pain and pressure and govern the sense of touch. They also sense temperature, advising the brain when it's time to slip on a sweater or change into shorts. Furthermore, the dermis is home to sweat glands, which help regulate body temperature by producing cooling perspiration. Blood vessels constrict to conserve body heat when you're cold, along with their usual duties of providing nourishment to all of the skin and its various structures.

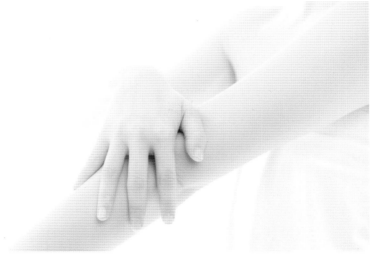

The third and innermost tier of the skin is called the subcutaneous layer. Mostly made up of fat, it provides insulation and protects bones and organs from bumps and bangs.

## How Diabetes Affects Your Skin

High blood sugar can rough up smooth skin in several ways. Elevated glucose results in high levels of compounds called advanced glycosylation end products (AGEs), which damage nerves and blood vessels that are necessary to keep skin healthy. However, your body's defense against high blood sugar may cause collateral damage to the epidermis, as you'll read in a moment. The first two major conditions we'll discuss, dry skin and skin infections, are common medical problems that can affect anyone, whether they have diabetes or not. However, people who have the disease are far more likely to develop these skin conditions. Many of the lesser-known skin problems discussed later primarily afflict people with diabetes.

## Dry Skin

If you spend all day scratching and your skin would make an iguana blush, chances are you're going to flunk your next blood-sugar test. When glucose levels rise too high, the body tries to get rid of the excess sugar through frequent urination. The more you urinate, the more fluid your body loses. If you don't replace that

## Gum Disease: Nothing to Smile About

You may not think of the moist tissue that lines the inside of your mouth as skin, but it is. And, like your external covering, the skin inside your pie hole can become infected. In fact, having diabetes is one of the leading risk factors for gum disease, which is also known as periodontal disease. Bacteria in the mouth can infect the gums, causing inflammation known as gingivitis. Left untreated, the problem can deteriorate to periodontitis, or the breakdown of bone and tissue that hold your choppers in place, resulting in lost teeth. Studies show that diabetes patients who don't maintain tight glucose control have an especially high risk for periodontal disease. In addition to keeping blood sugar under control, brushing and flossing at least twice a day and seeing your dentist for cleanings and checkups on a regular basis can help you keep your smile

lost fluid by guzzling lots of water, you become dehydrated, which causes (among other symptoms) dry skin.

As skin loses moisture, it becomes itchy. In severe cases, red scales may form. Scratching can cause sores to crack, opening the skin to an invasion of infectious bacteria. (See Skin Infections on the next page.) Damage to blood vessels and nerve endings in the skin from high glucose levels makes matters worse.

Of course, you don't need diabetes to develop dry skin. But people with diabetes need to be particularly wary of the environmental influences that can turn anyone's skin to parchment. In cold

climates, winter is a worrisome time, since heating systems sap the air of indoor humidity and cold winds chap the skin. Hot showers or baths with soaps and shampoos strip protective sebum from the skin any time of year.

To prevent dry skin, follow these tips.

**Shorten your showers.** Long, hot showers or baths may feel great, but they strip away natural oil that keeps skin soft and moist. Bathe in warm water, use mild soap and shampoo, and don't linger too long. Pat yourself dry with a towel. And don't overdo it: Cleanliness may be next to godliness, but bathing too frequently will dry your skin.

**Stay well lubed.** Apply skin moisturizer after you bathe. Ask your doctor to recommend a brand. Slather the stuff on liberally everywhere except between the toes, which should be kept dry to avoid the fungal infections.

**Drink up.** Water, that is, to keep your body well hydrated.

**Get misty.** Unless you live in a tropical climate, use a humidifier to keep the air in your home and workplace from becoming dry during cold winter months.

# Skin Infections

Skin infections can afflict anyone, too, but doctors agree that having diabetes greatly increases the risk for an invasion of microscopic meanies. The bacteria called *Staphylococcus aureus* (better known as staph) and the fungus *Candida*

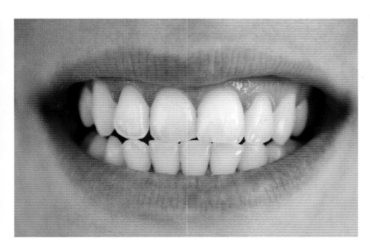

*albicans* cause many of the skin infections that are most common among people with diabetes.

Some of the more common bacterial skin infections to watch out for include these:

**Boils.** (Warning: The following definition gets pretty icky, fast.) Boils are painful red lumps that usually occur when bacteria infect a hair follicle. As inflammation worsens, the boil fills with pus and forms a yellow head before rupturing and draining. (Told you so.) Any part of the skin can develop a boil, although these ghastly little sores seem to like hairy areas, for obvious reasons, especially where you sweat a lot. (That means that the face, neck, armpits, and other sweat-inducing zones are most likely to get "boiled.") Hot compresses may relieve pain and make a boil heal faster. If a painful boil persists, see a doctor, who may drain the sore and give you a prescription for antibiotics. Above all, don't squeeze or pop a boil, which could worsen an infection.

**Carbuncles.** When a bunch of boils gang together, they form a carbuncle. Because they are more serious than single boils, you should see a doctor.

# A Scary Fungus Among Us

Fungal infections usually produce itchy, uncomfortable, and aesthetically displeasing skin rashes. But people with diabetes have a heightened risk for becoming infected with a potentially deadly fungus that causes a condition called mucormycosis (sometimes called zygomycosis). The problem starts with a common fungus from the class known as phycomycetes, which is found in soil and dying plants. Most people encounter this fungus every day without worry. But anyone whose immune system isn't working at full power—including patients with poorly controlled diabetes—may be vulnerable to these germs. Mucormycosis usually begins as a sinus infection, but inflammation may spread to the brain, lungs, or heart, resulting in blood clots or pneumonia. Mucormycosis can afflict the gastrointestinal tract, skin, and kidneys, too.

Symptoms may include:
* sinusitis (nasal discharge, with pain, pressure, or tenderness in the sinus region)
* fever
* swollen or protruding eyes
* scabs in the nasal passage
* red skin around the nose
* coughing or vomiting, especially if it produces blood
* shortness of breath
* abdominal pain
* pain in the flank, or lower back beneath the rib cage

Mucormycosis is a serious condition that requires immediate medical attention. Contact your physician if these symptoms develop and persist.

**Sties.** A sty is like a boil, only it forms on the edge of or under the eyelid. A sty may be painful or grow large enough to block vision. Warm compresses may relieve pain and encourage a sty to shrink, but see a doctor if the problem persists. Antibiotic creams can help heal a sty and prevent recurrence. Never squeeze or pierce a sty.

Some of the more common fungal infections (also known as tinea corporis) to afflict people with diabetes include these related conditions:

**Athlete's foot.** You don't have to be a jock to get this itchy, scaly menace. (You can read more about it on page 175.)

**Jock itch.** Likewise, you don't have to wear an athletic supporter to develop this uncomfortable condition, though those snug-fitting protective garments can contribute to the problem (which explains why jock itch usually afflicts males). Also known as tinea cruris, the problem begins as an itchy red rash around the genitals, which can spread to the inner thigh.

**Ringworm.** As the name suggests, this fungal infection forms ring-shape scales on the skin that may itch. (Fortunately, it doesn't mean you have worms, though having an infectious fungus is nothing to brag about.) Ringworm often develops on the scalp, though it can turn up on other parts of the body. Ringworm of the toenails and fingernails, called onychomycosis, is a common problem. The nails turn thick and discolored, and there's not much your manicurist can do about it.

Fungal infections can turn up on other parts of the body, too. Over-the-counter medications may help, but your physician can prescribe a more powerful antifungal drug to clear up persistent problems.

So take steps to prevent skin infections.

**Keep it clean.** We know, we know, we just got done telling you that bathing too often can worsen dry skin. But that doesn't mean you should turn into Pigpen. A thorough daily cleaning will keep bacteria at bay.

**Keep it dry.** Again, isn't dry skin a threat? Yes, but so are dark, damp places on the body, such as between the toes and under the arms, where fungus can grow. Using a little talcum powder on areas where skin rubs against skin isn't a bad idea.

# More Skin Problems

The following conditions are less common than dry skin and skin infections (some are downright rare). Some are merely cosmetic problems, while others produce physical symptoms. Recognizing them can help you get prompt medical attention and prevent needless worry.

**Acanthosis nigricans (AN).** This condition produces thick, dark patches on the body; doctors sometimes say the skin appears velvety. The armpits, back, neck, and other regions prone to sweating are most often afflicted. AN may occur because an unknown "trigger" in the body causes skin cells to accumulate. Some doctors believe excess insulin is one potential trigger, which may be why AN appears to be more common in people with type 2 diabetes. In fact, while AN doesn't hurt or itch, it's a signal to doctors that a patient may have insulin resistance. (A rare form of AN has been linked to cancerous tumors.) Given its association with type 2 diabetes, it's no surprise that AN is more common in obese people; it also seems to be more prevalent in people with dark skin.

**Diabetic blisters.** Sometimes called bullosis diabeticorum, this uncommon problem is most likely to afflict someone with diabetic neuropathy, or nerve damage that is caused by elevated blood sugar levels. Blisters, like those you might get from a serious burn, may form on the hands, fingers, arms, legs, feet, or toes. Although they are usually painless, diabetic blisters may be alarming.

If you get one, though, don't worry too much; they will usually heal on their own, especially if you get your blood sugar under control.

**Diabetic dermopathy.** This common diabetes-related skin problem is also known as "shin spots," since the spots usually appears on the front of the lower legs. The shiny round or oval brown spots develop as tiny blood vessels in the legs narrow and thicken. Shin spots are usually harmless other than mild itching or burning, so they don't require treatment.

**Diabetic thick skin.** No one likes being called "thin skinned," but your doctor isn't paying you a compliment if he or she says your skin is thick. It's not clear why, but diabetes patients tend to have thicker-than-average hides. The problem can take one of several forms. In digital sclerosis, the digits in question are the fingers and toes, but this term includes the back of the hands, too. The skin not only thickens; it turns waxy-looking and feels tight. The joints may stiffen, too. When the skin on the back of the neck or upper back thickens, doctors call the problem scleroderma diabeticorum. Lotions or moisturizers may help soften the skin.

**Disseminated granuloma annulare.** Similar in appearance to necrobiosis lipoidica diabeticorum (see below), this condition causes a ring-shape rash that is red, brown, or sometimes simply a slightly different shade than one's skin. It can spring up on the trunk, neck, arms, legs, and even ears. If the rash is hidden from sight, you may not require any treatment, since it doesn't ache or itch. To treat the condition for cosmetic purposes, doctors usually prescribe steroids.

**Eruptive xanthomatosis (EX).** As the name suggests, eruptive xanthomatosis creates bulging deposits of yellowish fat in the skin. The thinner the skin, the more noticeable the eruption, which is why the eyelids are so commonly affected (a problem doctors call xanthelasma). However, EX can pop up in other parts of the body, particularly the buttocks. In addition to itching, the lumpy skin is usually rimmed in red. This is not many people's idea of an attractive look, but EX is more than a cosmetic concern. These skin eruptions form when unhealthy levels of fats called triglycerides build up in the blood because the body has become resistant to insulin and cannot get rid of them. In other words, lumpy skin may be the least of your worries. Treatment consists of eating a healthy diet and taking medication to control glucose and blood fats.

**Necrobiosis lipoidica diabeticorum (NLD).** This rare condition produces blotches on the skin, too, in the form of large, reddish-brown, scarlike sores. Over time, the sores may turn yellow. NLD can be itchy and painful. (Patients without diabetes may develop the condition, in which case doctors just call it necrobiosis lipoidica.) NLD is three times more common in women than in men. No one knows what causes the condition. It appears to occur as collagen (fiber that holds cells together) breaks down beneath the skin. There is no treatment for NLD, but if a sore breaks open, it requires prompt medical attention.

**Vitiligo.** Certain diseases, including type 1 diabetes, seem to predispose people to developing this harmless but cosmetically bothersome skin condition. Like type 1 diabetes, vitiligo is an autoimmune disorder, meaning it occurs when the body's immune system mistakenly attacks healthy cells. In this case, the victims are melanocytes, cells that make skin pigment. Vitiligo produces pale patches of discolored skin. The hands, arms, and other parts of the body that receive a lot of sun exposure are most commonly affected, although any portion of your epidermis is vulnerable.

**Yellow skin.** No one is certain why, but people with diabetes occasionally develop a yellowish hue to their skin and nails. According to one theory, the problem occurs because some varieties of those irksome advanced glycosylation end products (AGEs) we talked about earlier are yellow in color. If your glucose isn't under control, AGEs accumulate in the blood, which may tint the skin. Although having jaundiced skin is no fun, there is no treatment other than regaining control over blood sugar.

# APPENDIX A:
# Carb Exchange List

## 1 Vegetable Exchange
(5 grams carbohydrate) equals:

| | |
|---|---|
| ½ cup | Vegetables, cooked (carrots, broccoli, zucchini, cabbage, etc.) |
| 1 cup | Vegetables, raw, or salad greens |
| ½ cup | Vegetable juice |

## 1 Milk Exchange
(12 grams carbohydrate) equals:

| | |
|---|---|
| 1 cup | Milk: fat-free, 1% fat, 2%, or whole |
| ¾ cup | Yogurt, plain nonfat or low-fat |
| 1 cup | Yogurt, artificially sweetened |

## 1 Meat Exchange
(0 grams carbohydrate) equals:

| | |
|---|---|
| 1 ounce | Beef, pork, turkey, or chicken |
| 1 ounce | Fish fillet (flounder, sole, scrod, cod, etc.) |
| 1 ounce | Tuna or sardines, canned |
| 1 ounce | Shellfish (clams, lobster, scallops, shrimp) |

| | |
|---|---|
| ¾ cup | Cottage cheese, nonfat or low-fat |
| 1 ounce | Cheese, shredded or sliced |
| 1 ounce | Lunch meat |
| 1 whole | Egg |
| ¼ cup | Egg substitute |
| 4 ounces | Tofu |

## 1 Fruit Exchange
(15 grams carbohydrate) equals:

| | |
|---|---|
| 1 small | Apple, banana, orange, or nectarine |
| 1 medium | Peach |
| 1 | Kiwi |
| ½ | Grapefruit or mango |
| 1 cup | Berries, fresh (strawberries, raspberries, blueberries) |
| 1 cup | Melon, fresh, cubes |
| 1 slice | Melon, honeydew or cantaloupe |
| ½ cup | Juice (orange, apple, or grape) |
| 4 teaspoons | Jelly or jam |

# 1 Starch Exchange

(15 grams carbohydrate) equals:

| | |
|---|---|
| **1 slice** | Bread (white, pumper-nickel, whole-wheat, rye) |
| **2 slices** | Bread, reduced-calorie or "lite" |
| **¼ (1 ounce)** | Bagel, bakery-style |
| **½** | Bagel, frozen, or English muffin |
| **½** | Bun, hamburger or hot dog |
| **1 small** | Dinner roll |
| **¾ cup** | Cold cereal |
| **⅓ cup** | Rice (cooked), brown or white |
| **⅓ cup** | Barley or couscous, cooked |
| **⅓ cup** | Legumes (dried beans, peas, lentils) |
| **½ cup** | Beans, cooked (black or kidney beans, chick peas) |
| **½ cup** | Pasta, cooked |
| **½ cup** | Corn, potato, or green peas |
| **3 ounces** | Potato, baked, sweet or white |
| **¾ ounce** | Pretzels |
| **3 cups** | Popcorn, air-popped or microwaved |

# 1 Fat Exchange

(0 grams carbohydrate) equals:

| | |
|---|---|
| **1 teaspoon** | Oil (vegetable, corn, canola, olive, etc.) |
| **1 teaspoon** | Butter |
| **1 teaspoon** | Margarine, stick |
| **1 teaspoon** | Mayonnaise |
| **1 Tablespoon** | Margarine or mayonnaise, reduced-fat |
| **1 Tablespoon** | Salad dressing |
| **1 Tablespoon** | Cream cheese |
| **2 Tablespoons** | Lite cream cheese |
| **⅛** | Avocado |
| **8 large** | Black olives |
| **10 large** | Green olives, stuffed |
| **1 slice** | Bacon |

# APPENDIX B:
# Glycemic Index of Common Foods

## BREAD/CRACKERS

Bagel ...............................................72

Graham crackers............................74

Hamburger bun ............................61

Kaiser roll......................................73

Pita bread ......................................57

Pumpernickel bread.......................51

Rye bread, dark .............................76

Rye bread, light .............................55

Saltines...........................................74

Sourdough bread ...........................52

Wheat bread, high-fiber ................68

White bread ...................................71

## CAKES/COOKIES/MUFFINS

Angel food cake..............................67

Banana bread..................................47

Blueberry muffin ...........................59

Chocolate cake ..............................38

Corn muffin...................................102

Cupcake with icing.........................73

Donut ............................................76

Oat bran muffin .............................60

Oatmeal cookie ..............................55

Pound cake ....................................54

Shortbread cookies .........................64

## CANDY

Jelly beans ......................................80

Lifesavers........................................70

M&M's, peanut .............................33

Milky Way Bar ..............................44

## CEREALS/BREAKFAST

All-Bran .........................................42

Bran flakes......................................74

Cheerios .........................................74

Cocoa Krispies ...............................77

Corn flakes.....................................83

Cream of wheat..............................70

Frosted Flakes.................................55

Golden Grahams ............................71

Grape Nuts.....................................67

Life.................................................66

Oatmeal .........................................49

Pancakes .........................................67

Puffed Wheat .................................67

Raisin Bran ....................................73

Rice Bran .......................................19

Rice Krispies ..................................82

Shredded Wheat.............................69

Special K ........................................66

Total................................................76

Waffles ...........................................76

## DAIRY

Chocolate milk...............................34

Ice cream, vanilla...........................62

Ice cream, chocolate .......................68

Milk, skim.....................................32

Milk, whole...................................27

Soy milk......................................30

Yogurt, low-fat ..............................33

## FRUITS/JUICES

Apple ..........................................38

Apple juice ...................................41

Apricot........................................57

Banana ........................................55

Cantaloupe....................................65

Cherries........................................22

Cranberry juice ..............................68

Dates.........................................103

Fruit cocktail .................................55

Grapefruit ....................................25

Grapefruit juice ..............................48

Grapes.........................................46

Orange ........................................44

Orange juice..................................52

Peach..........................................42

Pear ...........................................37

Pineapple .....................................66

Pineapple juice ..............................46

Plum ..........................................39

Raisins.........................................64

Watermelon...................................72

## LEGUMES

Baked beans ..................................48

Black beans ...................................30

Black-eyed peas ..............................42

Chick peas.....................................33

Fava beans ....................................79

Lentils, red ...................................25

Lima beans ...................................32

Peas, dried ...................................22

Pinto beans....................................45

Red kidney beans ............................19

## PASTA

Fettuccini .....................................32

Gnocchi .......................................68

Linguini .......................................55

Macaroni......................................45

Macaroni & cheese..........................64

Ravioli w/meat ...............................39

Spaghetti ......................................41

Spaghetti, wheat .............................37

## RICE/GRAIN

Brown rice ....................................55

Couscous.......................................65

Instant rice ...................................87

Long-grain rice...............................56

Risotto ........................................69

Vermicelli.....................................58

## SNACK FOODS

Corn chips ...................................74
Granola bar ...................................61
Peanuts...................................15
Popcorn...................................55
Potato chips...................................54
Pretzels...................................81
Rice cakes...................................77

## SOUPS

Black bean...................................64
Lentil ...................................44
Minestrone...................................39
Split pea ...................................60
Tomato ...................................38

## SUGARS/SPREADS

Honey...................................58
Strawberry jam ...................................51

## VEGETABLES

French fries ...................................75
Potato, baked ...................................85
Potato, mashed...................................91
Carrots, boiled ...................................49
Carrots, raw ...................................16
Corn, sweet ...................................55
Peas...................................48
Sweet potato...................................44